THE
ENERGY DIET

Boost your energy, Become happy, Lose weight

Michele Murray

This book is dedicated to Rose and Dean; the reasons I need energy, and the loves of my life.

Table of Contents

THE ENERGY DIET

Imagine this scenario. You're lying in bed. You're in a deep sleep and the alarm starts going off. You jump at the sound, while simultaneously trying to hit the snooze button. You accidentally hit the dismiss button, and now you've overslept. You get up in a panic. You're still exhausted and hazy and now find yourself in a panicked rush. Your kids aren't listening, and you find yourself screaming loud enough for the entire neighborhood to hear. You search for a clean coffee cup, but your spouse didn't unload the dishwasher, and you are filled with rage. You pour the kids some sugary cereal and stuff a piece of toast and jam in your own mouth before yelling at everyone to get their shoes on and get in the car.

You get to work late as usual and offer a weak hello and a nod to your boss who just happens to strolling past your desk as your scurry. Could you be imagining it or did your boss just give you a weird look? You panic. "Oh God, I'm going to be fired." You sit at your desk worrying about it for the next three hours and, therefore, get absolutely nothing done. Lunchtime comes, and you crave comfort food. You rush to car and head to the drive through. After wolfing down a huge cheeseburger, some fries, and a big caffeinated soda, you're back at work. The boss seems fine now, you worried for nothing. However, as the 2 o'clock sleepies set in, you can hardly keep your eyes open.

"Okay, I'd better go get a caramel latte to try to stay awake here or I really will be in trouble," you say silently. After an afternoon that stretched on forever, you finally get to leave and go home. You are getting a little energy back, but you just really can't be bothered with cooking tonight. Not after that long day. You're just wrecked. You pick the kids up and they are moaning and whining; one seems to just be bouncing around in the backseat for some reason. "What is wrong with these children? Omg!" Your head feels as if it is going to explode.

You get home and, since you have no groceries, you jump online to order a few pizzas. You choose the cinnamon pizza for dessert. Once the pizza is done and eaten, you realize that you need to get the kids' homework finished. As they sit at the table struggling to get homework done, you wonder why they can't just sit and focus? After a painfully long hour of nagging them to finish their papers, you trudge upstairs to get everyone ready for bedtime. All of the sudden everyone seems to have spurts of energy. They're running all around. You seem to have gotten a second wind, so you harness this power to get everyone into bed and doors closed. They're not quiet, but at least they're in the rooms. So you call it a victory. You finally get to the couch. You should go to bed, but you're wide awake now from the sprints you just took up and down the hall from room to room. You can hear children moving around overhead, but you just can't be bothered to go up and handle it. It's midnight and you're still wide awake, even though you know you have to be up in six hours. You decide to go lay in bed, where you spend an hour looking at your phone before finally dozing off. Then the alarm starts its nagging. Here you go again....

Now imagine this scenario.

You are lying in bed. It's morning. The birds are chirping outside, and the first rays of sunshine are starting to stream through your windows. Your eyes slowly flutter awake. Your sense of consciousness quickly comes into focus. You easily sit up, no pains, no sore necks, no grubby eyes. You feel rested and in a good mood. You sit on the edge of the bed, give your arms and legs a good stretch to get the blood flowing, and set off to get your morning started. You have a nice, calm energy and feel ready to take on the busy day ahead. You go into the kitchen for breakfast but don't feel that hungry. So you just have a nice cup of coffee. Your kids aren't listening when you urge them to get dressed for the day. Still, you're able to get them on the right track with a few gentle reminders. You were up in time to prepare a healthy breakfast for the family.

You get to work and overhear your coworker saying something snarky about you. "Whatever," you think to yourself before moving on. At lunch you are hungry, but since you feel so light and airy today, you settle on a big, fresh salad because you know you won't feel guilty after eating it. Your afternoon seems to fly by once you get focused on that new project you're working on. All of a sudden it's time to clock out and go home. You stop at the grocery store on the way home and instead of loading the cart with sweets, crisps, sodas and junk, you pick up some fresh vegetables, a nice-looking cut of meat, and some colorful and juicy fruit.

You get home and have a nice evening with the kids doing their homework while you prepare a healthy meal for your family. After dinner and a cozy evening, you notice the children yawning, and you scoot them off to bed. You and your spouse get an hour or two to relax or get a few things done around the house before your eyes start to get heavy. You want to get a good night's sleep again, so you head to bed. Minutes after laying down, you are asleep. You are a superhuman. You kicked the ass out of life today. You are the best mom/dad/wife/husband/kid/friend/other in the world. Look at you go.

Do you ever have those days when you just wake up in a good mood, your body feels fresh and light, no aches and pains, no tired eyes, no hitting the alarm clock a dozen times? Your entire day just seems to go as planned? Nothing really stresses you out. Those are the best days.

***

Wouldn't it be great to have the second type of day each and every day—to wake up and have the energy you need to deal with life's challenges full of strength and not constantly trying to just make it through? A life without energy is a life unfulfilled. A life without energy is a life full of missed opportunities. A life without energy, is a life of unhappiness.

A life without energy is a life of unhappiness.

Why does it seem that so many of us struggle with having the right amount of energy to make it through the day? Is it the overburdened schedules, lack of sleep, or our overwhelmed mental facilities? Yes, those issues probably all contribute to our lack of energy. However, some people seem to be able to manage the same obligations, with the same hours in the day, and the same struggles in life with ease. What's their secret? Is life easier for those with unlimited amounts of energy stores? Undoubtedly so.

In this book, we tackle the biggest reason for the lack of energy in modern times, and that is our diet; what we eat. We have gone from eating a diet exclusively made up of real food (meats, seeds, nuts, fruit, and veg) to eating a diet mainly consisting of fake food (sugary, processed and refined carbohydrates, i.e., food substitutes). We all know that we need to eat healthier, stop eating so much sugar, stop eating fast food, and frozen meals, and yet, we can't. We are addicted to this fake food. I'm an engineer by trade, not a doctor and I'm writing this book as an engineer, somebody who figures out how to make systems function. What steps can we take to design a healthy lifestyle when there is so much resistance. I wanted to design a program that would let us go from eating addictive, energy sucking Fake Food to eating all Real food in a few simple steps. There are many proponents and naysayers for a bevy of diets. Some think the Keto Diet, where you eat loads of healthy fats, is the best. Some think a Vegan diet, where you eat nothing, but plants are the best. I don't know if there is a right answer to that debate, but I do know that if you can eat Real Food, all the time, without Fake Food mixed in, you are going to be bursting with energy, and way out ahead of the pack. Afterwards, you can fine tune what real foods work best for your body, but until you break your addiction to the Fake Food, you are not able to decide which type of diet works best for you. So, this book, will take you through the baby steps to make the switch, and make it as easy as possible. We use psychological tricks, biohacks, and self-training techniques to make sure that once we hack, we never go back. So, let's get started.

Introduction

You are about to change your life. Let's not underestimate this important moment in time. Once you learn the new way of thinking introduced in this book, you won't be able to go back to living the way you are now. We are going to rewire your brain, change the way you view food, and start you on the path to a long and healthy life. Not only are you going to be a new person, but you are going to spread this knowledge to those you love. You will slash your children's risk of being diagnosed with childhood diabetes, your entire family will be calmer and even-keeled because of this big change you are going to make. You are going to successfully reroute your entire trajectory and that of your family. Let's get into this momentous occasion.

This isn't a normal diet book. When I use the word *diet* in the title, I am not referring to losing weight and fitting into size two skinny jeans in three weeks. When we talk about diet in this book, it is simply defined as "what we eat." Our intent is to get away from associating food with weight, and instead associate it with feel good triggers such as energy, happiness, and power.

Before we start, I'll let you in on a little bit about my own journey to living life full of energy and show why I'm such a proponent of food being used as a boost in today's modern world. I grew up in the eighties and nineties, the decades which saw a marked upswing in which fast food drive throughs were on every corner, food bought in the grocery store came out of a cardboard box or plastic container, and fresh vegetables and fruit were expensive, time consuming and easily missed. Very similar to what we see today.

We lived in a little suburb in Southern California where the women were modern, the men were shaggy and we played out in the sunshine year-round. I remember hitting up Taco Bell, McDonalds, Jack in the Box, In-N-Out, and Carl's Jr. a few times a week. With my parents both working, we would get picked up from daycare and rotate the drive thrus just so we had enough time to get home, get our homework done, and get into bed. On the nights my mom did cook, we'd eat things like Swanson's frozen dinners, and mac and cheese with hotdogs mixed through swallowed down with some Little Hug (fake) Fruit Barrels, or Soda, or chocolate milk if we were being a bit healthy. Every once in a while, we'd have some vegetables thrown in on the side, and each time, my brother and I would act like Mom was trying to make us eat live bugs. Tears and tantrums would ensue, followed by having to sit at the table for hours until every last bite of that disgusting vegetable was choked down. Mom, being so traumatized at trying to get us to eat our vegetables, would resort back to Taco Bell the next evening. As you can imagine, after a long day's work, it was too much effort to go through that fiasco again.

My food life continued that way, until I got out on my own for college. I studied abroad in London and had my first experience living on my own and feeding myself. Not only did they not have most of my normal foods in London, but I was on a college student's budget. In order to survive, I did what any broke 18-year-old would do, I bought loads of instant noodles, white bread with peanut butter and jelly, and the big packs of Doritos. That got me through the semester without withering away, but I remember being exhausted the entire time. Here I was, the first time living on my own, in a big and glamourous city, and yet, I was napping all the time and missing out on so many experiences. I never even thought that my food choices might have been ruining such an epic experience.

I got back to California and moved into an apartment across the street from my college and got an internship at an engineering firm. I had a *little* more money in my pocket and was able to afford some of the finer offerings life had. So, back to fast food I went. I'd have a breakfast burger before class, a fried taco before heading to work and pick up a cheeseburger on the way home before I dove into my homework load. I was studying full time and working at a top firm, and just trying to stay on top of everything. The only problem was I could barely stay awake. I would sneak in naps at any chance, blow off assignments because I just didn't have the energy to sit up all night to get them done, sit at work with my eyes half-closed, just wishing I could lay down somewhere and go to sleep. I was completely exhausted. To add to it, I could feel my mood swings becoming worse and worse. There were quite a few times I just pulled over in my car, completely overwhelmed and cried my eyes out. I just couldn't understand how I was meant to accomplish everything, and all that made me want to do was sit down and do nothing. A severe bout of depression came on, and I eventually packed my things and flew to Australia for almost a year, just to get my head straightened out. While there I made some new friends and started doing a lot of fun things like hiking a few times a week, going to the beach after work for a swim every day, and eating the Australian way. Australians are known for their health-focused lives, and it's hard not to get sucked into that dynamic when you see all these bright-eyed, beautiful people running around (literally running—those people are machines) all the time.

When I got back to California this time, I was feeling good. I looked great, had a clear head, and was ready to get back to my real life. While I had all the motivation in the world, once I had gotten home, my old habits were quick to return, hurling me into another bout of serious depression. Thinking that the problem was

California, and not my lifestyle, that was making me sick, I once again up and left. My company had acquired a new office, and I was approved for a transfer. This time I was bound for the bright lights and wild nights of New York City. I got into the swing of city life quickly. Being single, employed and excited for life once again, I quickly made new friends and became a fixture on the nightlife scene. I adopted the cigarettes and champagne diet, so beloved by 20-something-year-olds in the city. I was out every night, sometimes until the morning, just trying to keep up in this new and exciting world. During the day, I'd be hungover, feeling like I was on death's door. I was beyond tired, felt like shit, looked like shit, and would just try to get through the workday, so I could go back out that night and start drinking again. The drinking would give me that hit of energy and make me feel a little bit better, only to have to wake up the next morning and do it all again. This cycle went on for years. I didn't have a clear mind, so was never forced to really examine how badly I was treating myself, and how much more difficult I was making my own life.

During this time, I met the love of my life and got married. One of the nights we had gotten home from partying, I asked him if it was time to have a baby. I was getting older and knew many friends who had tried to get pregnant and were having difficulties. I knew my lifestyle wasn't the healthiest and figured I would soon find myself in the same boat. As luck would have it, we got pregnant the first month. All the sudden, I went from years of going out every night, drinking, smoking, and eating crap to having to quit drinking, quit smoking, and quit my social life due to tiredness and being extremely annoyed by drunk people. I made all these huge changes within a week and, boy, was it tough. I was so emotionally and physically unprepared, feeling that I would have another few years to get to this stage. Every night I'd get home from work and find an entire evening stretched before me with no clue how to fill the time, extreme cravings for my old vices, and fear about what lay ahead. On a bit of a whim, I decided to start learning how to cook. My husband still jokes about when we first started dating, and I tried to make him a meal of steak and potatoes. The steak was still moo-ing at the table, and I had to call my mom to ask her how to boil the potatoes. If I was going to be a mom, I knew I'd need to change, and the first change would be to learn how to cook our meals.

Instead of going out partying, I'd spend my evenings cooking up new recipes I'd found online. While this was a great direction to go in, I'd be lying if I said I was making healthy meals. I was basically finding my favorite fast food and takeout foods and finding ways to make them at home. Though I'm not great at it, I learned to really love cooking. It made me relax and focus on something instead of worrying or feeling deprived of my old life. I soon discovered that if I put on an audio book, comedy show or podcast that cooking was even more enjoyable. After a short while, I grew to love it so much, that I went from eating out every meal, to cooking most of our meals at home, bringing leftovers for lunch, and picking more interesting options when we did eat out. I started feeling like fast food was too bland and didn't want to waste my time on something unless I found it extra delicious. While this was a great step to getting out of the fast food cycle, I didn't realize that cooking at home can be just as fattening (if not more) than eating out all the time. By the end of my pregnancy I had gained 60 pounds (my doctor was not pleased) and was swollen and aching in all directions. Not to mention, I was absolutely exhausted every waking moment of the day. Part of that was from being pregnant, but I was having difficulty being awake for most of the day. I'd get a spurt of energy in the evenings when it was time to cook, and then back to the couch to sit and eat my creation and fall asleep.

When my daughter was born, I was not prepared for just how overwhelming it would be. Up all night, having visitors nonstop, and just trying to recover for those first few months after the birth were extremely difficult. I had stopped cooking and was ordering take out for every meal. I was somehow even more tired than before, and I found myself just lying with her on the bed, crying and hoping she would go to sleep so that I could get a few moments of rest myself. I was constantly resentful of how stressful this experience was, how I didn't have anybody there with me during the day to help, and my body seemed to just feel worse, every passing day. After a few months of suffering, I went for a checkup at the doctors and was diagnosed with Post Partum Depression. I can't say I was that surprised. After dealing with depression so many times in my past, I felt I should have known that I would be one to come down with this horrible illness. However, this time was different. I wasn't depressed in the same way as before, this wasn't a sad and numb state of affairs, but an unhinged and rage-filled walk through hell. The doctor dosed me up with some pills and sent me on my way, advising me to see a therapist.

After a long spell of drugs and trying to get out and following my therapist's advice to meet other moms, I finally started feeling back to my normal self again. Not great, not terrible, but not in a constant state of angry, emotional panic. I started cooking again. This time, I was much more focused on learning to cook healthy food. Not only did I still have those sixty pounds of baby weight to lose, I also needed to learn how to feed a growing child. After a lot of time searching on the internet, I decided that the Atkins diet seemed to show the most promise of shedding the unwanted pounds quickly and I also liked most of the stuff on the list of foods to eat. The first day started off great. I was eating bacon, and microwaved pepperonis with melted cheese. Then some kielbasa for lunch, followed by a diet coke and whipped cream dessert. It wasn't bad at all. I stepped on the scale and was down five pounds by the end of the that first week. But, by God, by day three, the sugar cravings hit, and they hit hard. I went to my computer and tried finding recipes for low carb sweets. I'd put the baby in the stroller and set off to find special ingredients in a load of different grocery stores, trying to find all the alternate flours, the sugar substitutes, the low carb flours, just anything to make the sugar detox less difficult. I'd spend ages in the kitchen whipping up low carb cheesecakes, low carb cookies, and other fake desserts that would satisfy my sweet tooth but do nothing to kill the cravings. I went to the pharmacy and spent a fortune buying boxes of the different types of low carb candy bars, only to try them and be filled with disappointment. None of this was working, but I didn't give up hope. I bought loads of low carb dessert cookbooks hoping that there must be some miracle out there that would allow me to have my sweets and also lose the weight. All the while, I was very strict about not eating any fruit, and watching my vegetable intake closely to make sure I could have my treats and still not go over my carb limit for the day.

Eventually, as any avid dieter will tell you, the weight did come off. I was fearful of every bite I put in my mouth, still searching for tricks to consume sweet treats, and just as tired as ever, but that baby weight finally came off. Mostly. I was a few pounds over my pre baby weight, but it wasn't that noticeable, and I was a mom now, I was allowed a few extra pounds. As soon as I got back down to size, I ditched Atkins in a heartbeat. I hated being so restricted in my food choices, and I decided that as long as I was making my family meals consisting of whole foods, that would be good enough. As someone who has never loved vegetables, I decided that we needed to start eating more of those, and my, now toddler, was obsessed with berries, so we always had cartons of them in the fridge. I would sit and slave away in the kitchen all day, making big Sunday dinners every day of the week. Lots of whole foods, heavily buttered potatoes and veg, meat that was seasoned and seared perfectly, stews and pasta sauces that would simmer on the stove all day. We'd still eat out a few times a week, but I'd plan and prep beautiful dinners that I felt very impressed with. It was beautiful. I was proud of going from an emotional wreck party girl, to a healthy mom trying to do the best for her family. I started feeling good, and wanting to go for walks, wanting to go out and take my little family around to see things and spend quality time together. This was all new to me and I enjoyed the changes I saw taking place.

A few years later, my husband and I made the decision that we'd move to Ireland before my daughter started school. We moved from New York City to a small town in the country, where we could have a simple little life, and he could still commute to Dublin for work. I went from having a tiny little kitchen in our tiny little apartment to a huge kitchen with an island, in a massive house, with a car. In NYC I had grown accustomed to having my groceries delivered, my toilet paper delivered, toys delivered. Everything I bought was through my phone and placed at my door. Now, I had to go to the store for food, I had to go to multiple stores depending on what I needed. This was a whole new experience. Add onto it, that there weren't a million restaurants that delivered, there were two. Chinese and pizza. Neither of them particularly good. There were two fast food joints in town, and both required a little drive to reach. Mac and cheese wasn't to be found in the grocery aisles, and the same went for my other favorite treats and sweets. After a few trips to the grocery store I also realized that even if I decided to cook every meal, the ingredient selection was much smaller than I was used to. There were no tomatillos to be found. Fresh spices were limited to basil, parsley, dill, and cilantro. It was tough going for my newfound foodie desires. The upside was that it was very easy to find grass-fed meat and dairy, and the produce was beautiful and full of flavor, compared to most stores in the states.

Quite by accident, I had started eating a diet of whole, unprocessed foods. One day, seemingly out of nowhere, I realized that my energy levels were increasing steadily. It took a while, but when you go from being tired all the time, to feeling like you can get through the day without a nap; you notice. I started adding in little hikes during the week when my daughter was at school. I used the same technique as I did for cooking. I saved special podcasts or books for my hikes through the amazing forests of Ireland. That feeling of clear-headed invigoration, started to become a drug for me. I wanted to feel that way all the time. Every once in a while, we would go out to one of the fast food places, or happen upon a store that sold Mac and Cheese or Pop Tarts that I'd buy up. Every time, I'd eat these foods, I'd immediately feel crappy again. I started noticing the correlation of my diet to how I felt, energy wise. Like clockwork, if I ate Fake Food, within a few hours my energy levels would plummet. My emotions would start swinging, and I'd need a nap. Sensing that there was a connection between what I ate and how my days played out, I started researching the relationship.

It took me years to fully quit my addiction to the processed food products that overwhelm our society. I tried to circumvent the inevitable at every turn, and would end up tired, moody and on the edge of depression. One day, I decided it was time to quit.

Notice the word "decide." Decide isn't an iffy word. When you decide to do something, that's it. Through hell or high water, you are going to make it work. It's very important to approach your decision to change with resolve. Don't allow yourself to waffle about and second guess your choices. You know in your gut that eating real food over fake food will make you feel better, you just have to figure out how to make the change. Luckily, I have designed a system for you, so that you don't have to spend years trying to figure it out. But, before we start, take a few moments and really *decide* that you want energy, that you want health, and that you want a happy life. Once you make that decision, you just need to follow the path and you will get there.

That's why I wrote this book. I read so many fabulous books about health, energy, diet, exercise, neurology, and more, and I wanted to put out an easy resource for those who need a helping hand with how to change their life to one of happiness, energy and purpose, but aren't quite sure where to start. Use this book as a friend, somebody that encourages you and gives you ideas when you're feeling frustrated and unmotivated. I have taken my engineering background and designed a step by step guide on how to transition from a diet full of sugar, processed foods and refined carbohydrates, and turn yourself into a lover of whole, real, and healthy foods. Not only will you learn to love Real Food, but I've designed a program to help you transform your life in a few simple steps. This is not a medical book, it's not a book filled with scientific studies, it's not written by a doctor, it's not been studied. It's just helpful advice to be experimented with, put into practice, and tweaked for your own needs. Nobody knows you, like you.

THIS IS NOT MEDICAL ADVICE. PLEASE ASK YOUR DOCTOR BEFORE STARTING ANY NEW DIETS.

Why Diets Fail

If you've ever attempted a diet (or twelve of them), you might have wondered why it's so hard to stick to a diet plan. We have a general idea of what's healthy and not; we have a general idea of what makes us gain or lose weight. It's not that we lack motivation in wanting to be healthy. If I offered you a million dollars or a new body and lifestyle where you enjoyed healthy eating, looked great, and felt full of life, I'd bet a lot of you would take the healthy life; at the very least, you'd have a hard time deciding. We are all capable of having the lifestyle tomorrow; why don't we do it?

When we diet, what are our motivations? We may say health, and mean it, but most of us want to look good. Let's just be honest here. It would be great to feel better, our doctors might be nagging us about medical problems, but we are a vain species, and we mostly want to walk around looking slim and unjudged. We we think of being skinny as the answer to many of life's problems. Fixing health problems or thwarting future catastrophes are an added benefit, but that's not the reason most people try to overhaul what they eat. So, we start the diet off fast and furious. We make huge changes all at once and really give it our all. We lose some weight, get encouraged, and then might even kick it up a notch. We start buying all the fancy food items that our latest diet requires, push through all the temptations, and eagerly step on the scale to watch the number go down and down and down. Then, we hit the dreaded plateau. The weight stops coming off. We get frustrated. We remind ourselves of what losers we are, and this state of mind pushes back towards our old ways. So, we give up.

When your diet fails, your brain starts trekking down the familiar path of old feelings and you feel defeated. The feelings are so shameful that we turn to the one thing that always brings us comfort, food. Of course, it's the food we've been torturing ourselves with for months, so we indulge. The guilt suddenly floods over us, and it's just so miserable and uncomfortable, that we give up all together. Another diet failure, like every other time. Sound familiar?

We need to shift our entire mindset away from weight loss. Why? Well, weight loss takes a while, and if we are focusing on our weight, then when we get off track, the scale doesn't move (or worse, moves back up), our brains just find it very difficult to process as anything but a failure. This is so demotivating and uncomfortable, that our brains go into self-preservation mode. They'd rather us avoid the bad feelings altogether, so you and your brain decide to quit, rather than have to face those terrible thoughts again.

When we eat and only think of numbers, whether its calorie counting, or numbers on a scale, it's too difficult to maintain the motivation it requires to make the changes we need to make. Not only that, but when we link our diet to weight loss, the end goal is always far off in the future. It's too far away to overcome the daily hurdles of making these life changes. People are much more motivated by instant gratification, not some far off goal. Let's imagine a retirement plan. We keep putting money away, not knowing if we will ever see the payoff. If your company didn't take it out before your check made its way into your hands, would you even have a retirement account? Maybe. But it's hard to be motivated by something so far in the future, even if we know it's good for us, and something we need to do. A diet that is about weight loss is of the same mindset. You're giving up something you love (money or food), for some goal in the future(lots of money or a sexy bod), and we don't even know exactly what that goal looks like (how much will you have saved?/How will you actually look?). This is not a great structure for motivation.

Now, if I said, screw waiting, if you eat this salad for lunch, you will be slim this afternoon. Well, now we have some motivation to eat healthy right? I mean, you'd be a fool to say no to that deal. You'd never be so motivated to eat a salad in your entire life. You'd be cramming it down your gullet as quick as possible. When you receive a tangible reward in a short time frame, it's much easier to repeat the behaviour. We like to think of ourselves as entities completely separated from animals, but fortunately for us, our brains still behave in the same way, whether training a dog, or a human. Instead of feeling high and mighty, you can use this knowledge to retrain your brain. Let's take this structure of motivation and use it to achieve our goals. We aren't going to worry about losing weight. We are going to focus on whatever payoff we can get immediately from eating healthy. That's where we find our motivation to make this change. We have an immediate payoff. There is no greater way to make a new habit, than by immediately reinforcing the good you are doing.

So, how do we do this with our diet? Instead of focusing on weight loss, we focus on what we can immediately feel.

Energy.

How We Define Energy

Let's fine tune what we are talking about when we are discussing energy throughout the rest of this book. Energy as defined by Google:

energy

/ˈɛnədʒi/

noun

the strength and vitality required for sustained physical or mental activity.

Let's break this down a bit. Energy is the strength that is necessary for ongoing physical AND mental activity. So, not just your body's vitality, but just as importantly, we need energy for our mental activity. Our body is a system, and one doesn't work without the other.

When we talk about energy in this book, we are discussing ways for our bodies to feel good and carry us through the day. We are also talking about our mental state. We don't want to be going through the day in a fog; we want to be alert and on point. This is just as important to us, if not more, as how our bodies look. The good news is that once we start making healthy changes, our bodies will naturally lose the weight it needs to lose, but for this book, we aren't going to focus on weight loss, because we know it doesn't work. In this book, we are going to focus on energy and know that a healthy body will naturally take the weight off if it is needed.

Unfortunately, we all know many people that have suffered from a variety of mental health issues. Let's look at a common affliction, depression. We probably know at least one person who has suffered from this brutal condition, if not personally having been affected. When a person is depressed, a well-meaning doctor will usually tell them to go out, get some fresh air, take walks, hang out with friends. You see, these small activities have helped a lot of people counteract their depression, and they seem to work well. There's just one problem. The last thing a depressed person wants to do, is get out of bed and take a walk, or socialize. They are depleted of energy, mentally, and their body then also becomes depleted of energy physically. It's hard for people who have never suffered from depression to understand just how difficult it is to do these normal, everyday tasks. What is a walk to most, is climbing Mount Everest for the depressed individual. They do not have the energy to do what they need to do to get better.

Now, when we are thinking about our own daily energy levels, they hopefully aren't as extreme. But they work the same way. When we have a good energy level, everything becomes much easier to do. If you have a happy buzz going on in your day, taking a walk sounds like a pleasant activity. If you are struggling to grasp enough energy to shower, a walk is the last thing you'd want to do. How are you meant to cook beautiful, healthy meals when you are having a tough time just getting the essentials done? You won't. You will go get fast food at a drive through because that requires very little energy. It's extremely difficult to accomplish any goals if your energy levels aren't right. On the other hand, when you are having a high energy day, you can clean the entire house, run errands, cook your meals, and still have time to go out and enjoy yourself. I think your mental energy state is the most important factor to well-being and health. If you don't have the mental energy, you are constantly fighting an uphill battle. If you can optimize your mental energy, then everything else becomes so much easier and manageable. In this book, we are going to find ways to hack our brain, initiate new habits and get, what I like to call, a **Happy Buzz**.

The Happy Buzz is the state of mind where we flow from one thing to the next with little aggravation, little motivation, and little effort. We want our diet to be a simple habit that we do effortlessly and enjoy—not a huge and daunting task we have to undertake. We will do this by introducing a new way of eating, little by little, until we have quit fake foods. Then we examine how to get our mental energy levels right and end with more ways to optimize your energy levels. The result being a happy, healthy, new you.

What to Eat

In order to find out what to eat to give us the most energy, I read through countless books and studies. I was looking to find common threads; foods everyone agreed were healthy and healing, regardless of what diet a person subscribed to. As anybody that has ever followed more than a couple of diet plans can attest to, it is near impossible to find a plan from a doctor/ nutritionist that hasn't been "debunked" by another well-meaning doctor/nutritionist. Some promote eating a plant-based vegan diet, which consists of an array of vegetables, fruit, no meats, or eggs or cheeses. If you can't give up cheese, you can become a vegetarian, which is similar to being a vegan but allows dairy. Another group promotes eating like a caveman (the Paleo Diet), eating only whole, unprocessed foods, except no dairy or starchy vegetables. Their diet consists mostly of meats, eggs, vegetables and nuts. Then you have a similar diet, the Keto diehards, who are kind of like the Paleo, but allow dairy. However, you have to drastically limit carbs, including vegetables, and focus on eating lots of natural, unprocessed fats. One doctor may recommend cutting out as much fat as possible, while another doctor thinks sugars and carbs are the bad guys, and to focus on cutting those down. Each of these popular diets have fanatical proponents, and just as many naysayers. The few studies on each diet can be swung to fit whichever argument is trying to be made. It's almost impossible for us to know, at this time, what the magic formula is for having the most healthy diet. So, what is a normal person to eat if they want to feel good and have the Happy Buzz energy?

I've come to realize that the easiest way to approach the conundrum of differing advice is to let your body be your guide. When we think of food in terms of energy, it becomes a lot easier to decide what to eat. White bread is universally looked down upon by nutritionists, but we don't really need to know the reasons why if we look at food as energy.

Experiment 1: Eat a Sandwich

Suppose you can have whatever type of sandwich you'd like in this experiment. Ham and cheese, peanut butter and jelly—it's up to you. What you are going to do is have your sandwich and set a timer. An hour after you've finished eating, I'd like you to note how you feel. Do you feel alert and clear headed with the Happy Buzz? Or do you feel like you need a place to lie down and take a nap?

White bread is a refined and highly processed carbohydrate. When you first eat it, it will cause a rise in blood sugar followed by a plunge in insulin levels leading to fatigue, tiredness, and lethargy. If a sandwich makes us feel terrible an hour later, why do so many of us have one for lunch every day? After eating it, we can barely keep our eyes open for the afternoon. This is a horrible energy plan. We have a slice of toast in the morning, and then have difficulty getting moving and starting the day.

When we start to look at foods in terms of energy, we don't need to focus on what we are allowed to eat, or what we are not allowed to eat. We are eating, simply, to give us a Happy Buzz energy to get through our days. Not even to just get through, we want to *enjoy* our days. It's almost impossible to enjoy anything if you are fatigued and weak. Well, you'd enjoy a nap at that point, but we can't live the life we want, if we are constantly longing for our bed. By contrast, if we have a stable energy level all day, we can accomplish so much, and do it with ease, all while enjoying our experiences.

Experiment 2: Drink a juice

Once again, this can be whatever type of juice you like, but it needs to be fresh, nothing from a carton in the grocery store. Bonus points if you get a juice made with a mix of vegetables and fruits. Drink the juice and pay attention to your body while drinking. If you really tune in, you can almost feel the nutrients hitting your bloodstream. It's a bit like cold streams of energy flooding out from your chest into other areas. You feel good after drinking that juice. You can actually feel your body wake up as it's going down. It's almost like your body was craving that high hit of vitamins and nutrients, and is having a little party in your bloodstream.

Now, I hope you don't take from these little experiments that I am saying to never eat a sandwich and live on juices. No. Juices are high in sugar from all the fruit, so you only want to have them once in a while. Although by the end of this process you probably won't be eating many sandwiches anymore, that isn't the point of the experiment. What we are taking from these experiments is the realization that what goes into our mouth determines how we feel during the day. Use food as a weapon against the energy suckers. Use food as your tool, not something to feel guilty or angelic about. You are in control. You are the one who either suffers or thrives, and you are a smart and in-control sort of person who chooses to thrive.

So, back to our first question: what does a person eat if he or she wants to feel good and have that Happy Buzz energy? Are you ready for the revelation? Are you ready for the big reveal and master diet plan? Okay, here it goes...

We simply eat food that gives us energy during the day, leaving the energy sucking food for the evening when it's almost time for bed, or eventually, not at all..

Real Food vs Fake Food

←———— \\ ————→

To make our lives a bit simpler and avoid having to test every single food item to see if it gives you energy, or drains your energy, I'm going to let you in on an easy way to make good food decisions. Now, when I tell you this secret, you will be gob smacked. I wish I could say it is because I am about to tell you the most clever idea you have ever heard. But sadly, no. I am about to tell you the most obvious and mundane thought in maybe the existence of the world. However, when I tell it to you, it will probably hit like a ton of bricks. We have been so brainwashed by the diet industry, that we have lost sight of a very basic rule when it comes to food. In fact, it's so obvious, that you might be annoyed at ever spending money on a diet book, or diet food. You ready for the big secret to healthy, energy and happiness?

Eat Real Food.

What is Real Food, you might ask? Real Food is any food that comes from the ground, the sea, or a pasture, and hasn't been messed with. It can't have been processed into another product, I.e., a potato being turned into potato chips. It doesn't come in a package with a Brand plastered across the front. It hasn't been modified by adding heaps of sugar to make it palatable. Real Food is a food that consists of one ingredient and can be easily identified as either a meat, seafood, a dairy product or produce. Chicken thighs, steak, shrimp, eggs, milk, bananas, cashews, beans, are just a few examples of Real Food.

Yes, there is a lot of debate about whether certain Real Foods are great for your waistline. Some diets warn against eating potatoes and bananas. Others don't think red meat is good for your heart. There are a lot of differing opinions on what is the best type of Real Food to eat for health. However, for this book, we are going to leave all that controversy to the side and revisit it later. Those ideas can be explored only after you have stopped eating Fake Food. In order to quit Fake Food, we aren't going to limit our Real Food options. As far as we are concerned, all Real Food is going to be better for your health and energy when compared to Fake Food. If you **need** a sweet treat, eating an apple is much better than eating cookies. Once you have beaten your Fake Food addiction, you will have the tools to fine tune your Real Food choices even further.

Fake Food Kills

Fake Food is an experiment imposed upon all of us, and it has failed. We only need to visit a grocery store to see how Fake Food has permeated our culture to a huge extent. If you think of your local shop, you only have one or two aisles consisting of Real Food. Usually off to one side, the aisles will have loads of produce and then a section with meat and seafood, and off to the side, the dairy area. Then, if you look out you might see another 15-20 aisles worth of Fake Food. Instant dinners, a cookie aisle, a chip aisle, a soft drink aisle... On and on it goes, with thousands of neat and tidy little packages of Fake Food sure to make the taste buds sing.

Fake Food has only existed for about a century. Up until that point, you'd have to go to your local butcher for meat. If you lived by the sea, you could visit a fishmonger for a fresh fish. Growing your own produce was the norm, and you would eat a vegetable and/or fruit with every meal. Long before our societies learned about agriculture, humans would spend their days hunting for wild animals or fishing. They would scour the landscape for edible plants to add into their diet. Our bodies are evolved to eat this type of food. When our bodies eat Fake Food, they don't know what to do with it. Don't know how to process it. The microbiome doesn't understand where to use it. Our entire system gets messed up. Most killer diseases of the modern era can be traced back to people eating Fake Food. Everything from heart attacks, to stroke, to diabetes all revolve around our diet, and our diet is laden with Fake Food.

We have to beat our addiction to Fake Food, not only for health reasons, but so that our bodies can function as well as possible. When we eliminate Fake Food and replace it with Real Food, our brains, gut microbiome and energy levels all start to function properly again. We start being able to feel when we are full, start to only eat when we need to, and our senses all start coming into stark focus.

I have a theory about Real Food, that will make sense once you hear it. Many people start a diet and once they start losing weight, they become evangelical about their new way of eating. They will tell everybody who will listen, about all the positive changes it has made in their lives. They are so excited about their new lease on life, and they just want to share it with the world. Now, I have seen dieters like this many times. But the funny thing is, usually they are all doing different diets. One might be a caveman champion; one might be eating Keto and trying to show you why high fat is the only way to go. Whatever the diet, you will find apostles eager to share the good word. While I don't doubt that the diet has completely changed their lives, I do think that it isn't the actual diet that has made such a difference. I don't think that debating the ratio between fat/protein/carbs is the main driver of these transformations. No, I think the big awakening comes from one thing that all those diets have in common. Those diets all demand the followers to stop eating Fake Food. It is that change that has the biggest impact on the dieters, not the specific rules that must be adhered to. Now, I'm not saying that one way of eating may not be better than another, but I am saying that switching from Fake Food to Real Food will be the most drastic change you can make in your life. And it will yield the biggest results.

So, all those diets work; but there is just one glaring problem. While it is a prerequisite to quit Fake Food, there are hardly any instructions for how to do so. It's almost assumed as a passing thought. In reality, this is the most difficult part of any diet. Why isn't there a long list of ways to help the dieters overcome their addiction? If we know that diets work, then why are there overweight people? It's because the addiction isn't dealt with properly. This book will set out the steps to overcome that addiction. It will teach you to rewire your brain, so you associate food with your energy levels, not weight and size. This is the missing link that has been overlooked for so long in our decades long fight against food related illnesses.

How to Use This Book

This book is broken into two parts. The first part goes through the basic steps to change your diet and lifestyle to maximize your energy levels. The steps have been designed in a way to make the transition from Fake Food to Real Food as easy as possible, and it is suggested to complete each step before moving onto the next. You will know you have completed the step when the step has become a habit, meaning you don't need to think about it. That step has become second nature to you. Once you have a good grip on the step, it is time to move on to the next. Remember that these are changes for life, so if it takes a little time to complete a step, the time is relatively short compared to a lifetime of being tired and.

The second part of this book is broken into chapters discussing extra ways to implement the steps and more ways to improve your energy levels even after you have completed the steps. Feel free to skip ahead to Part Two even while working through the steps. Use any and all combinations of tricks and hacks. Make the process easy for yourself by trying different techniques until one works well for you. Everybody is different, so while the steps will work for all, we can tailor the approach to play to our strengths.

PART ONE

THE STEPS

STEP 1:

One Fruit, One Veg and One glass of Water

←————\\————→

This may seem like an easy first step. That's good, because it's one of the easiest ways to get your energy levels up.

Cut the Coke

As countless studies show, there are a lot of people who fail to even drink a single glass of water every day. I personally know quite a few people who only drink soft drinks every day. We all know this isn't good for us. Soft drinks are full of sugar—a definite energy sucker. Soft drinks give you a shot of energy followed by a crash sparking the need for another to try and get your energy back up. This is not a Happy Buzz. This is more like a manic toddler who just ate a bag of pixie stix kind of a buzz. Then you have the diet soda drinkers who aren't ingesting the sugar water, but a fake sugar water. There is more and more information coming out about how the chemical sweeteners are just as dangerous as drinking the real sugar. However, we need to recognize that sodas are addictive, so it may not be easy to quit right away. If you are able to give them up and switch to water, then do it. If not, we can take it a step at a time, until you have phased soda out of your diet. All we need to do is start adding in water. Overtime, you will up the amount of water you drink and cut down on the soda. For example, the first week, you add in one glass of water each day. The second week add in a second glass, and so on and so on until you reach your eight glasses per day. Water gives you a refreshed and clean feeling in the body that will help your entire body function more easily, giving us more energy, and in turn feeling happier and healthier.

Produce

At the same time, we are going to add in some fruit and vegetables. Just as with water, there are many of us that don't eat any fresh fruit or vegetables in a typical day. Whatever your starting point, I want you to consciously add in one portion of fruit and one portion of vegetable each day. There was a famous study conducted by the University of Warwick that showed a direct "happiness benefit" for each extra daily portion on fruit and vegetables, up to eight portions per day. In our new mindset when dealing with food, we know that happiness directly correlates to energy. The more energy we have, the more we can focus on what matters, and the more we are able to accomplish, which will make us happier. This study shows that fruit and vegetables gave the 12,000 participants of the study a direct increase in "happiness." I believe that is because those extra nutrients and positive nutrition made their day easier and less stressed due to increased stable energy levels; they enjoyed the Happy Buzz.

Now, it's very difficult to go from a standard diet of lots of processed foods to eating eight portions of fruit and veg every day. So, once again, we are going to add it in slowly, trying to make the experience as fun as possible so that we enjoy the increased energy levels and start to enjoy healthy eating. We don't want to be holding our noses and shovelling in cabbage for the rest of our lives; we want to savour our food, bask in the sight of our colorful plate, and learn to appreciate nature's gift of these incredible edible plants. When you first start adding in fruits and veg, you want to take it slowly, for a number of reasons. You don't want to be overwhelmed with making too many changes at once. Also, if you don't eat a lot of fiber, eating eight servings of produce all the sudden will almost guarantee an unpleasant stomach situation.

So, we start with one extra serving of fruit and one extra serving of veg added to whatever you already eat. Fruit tends to be more easily consumed, just add in an apple at lunch time, or snack on some berries in the afternoon. Whatever your favorite fruit, buy that, eat that, just make sure you are adding it into your day. Vegetables can be a little trickier, because so many people believe themselves to not like vegetables. Coming from somebody who loves to cook, I understand that point. Vegetables get a bad rap because if they are prepared wrong, they can taste like garbage. Boil a carrot too long, and it will taste disgusting, whereas if you roast that carrot and put a sauce or beautiful seasoning on top, it will taste divine. Raw carrots might be boring on their own, but dip them into some well flavored hummus, tahini dip, dressing or just plain old table salt, and now you have an interesting snack. Don't worry about the calories of butter or olive oil, or even the salt content, just try to find ways to enjoy eating vegetables. Remember, we aren't focusing on weight loss, but energy and for the Happy Buzz to work, we aren't worrying about that, we are only worrying about getting more vegetables into our diet and retraining our taste buds to like the taste. So, eat your serving of fruit and then try out different types of recipes for the vegetable. If you try a new vegetable one way, say roasted, and you don't like it, try sautéing it next time. Season heavily with salt, pepper and any herbs and spices you happen to like. Try dips and sauces, gradually reducing the amount until you are just using it to flavor your already very tasty vegetable.

After a week of adding in one fruit and one vegetable, for the second week we will add two of each. The third week, add three servings of each, bearing in mind, that eventually we want 2-3 servings of fruit, and 5-6 servings of vegetables. So, in the fourth week, instead of adding another serving of fruit, you will be adding more vegetable. Go online and look at serving sizes for your produce, it's probably smaller than you think, and that vegetable you counted as one serving may actually have been enough to count as two. So, while 5-6 servings of vegetables may sound like a lot, in reality, you may only eat 2 different vegetables, but would just increase your portion size. Instead of one carrot, you'd eat three. Instead of a spoonful of broccoli, you'd fill up half your plate with it. Keep going in this direction until you have a solid intake of healthy produce every day, preferably eight servings if you can manage.

Brain Hacks

- Eat your fruit or veg at the start of your meal or snack. Allow yourself to eat whatever you'd like AFTER you finish the important part of eating your produce. During this step of our energy diet, if you want to stop at a fast food joint and pick up a double cheeseburger and fries, go right ahead. That's totally fine. However, before you bite into that burger, make sure you eat a salad, or a serving of broccoli, or carrots, or whatever vegetable you like. Eat that part first when you are at peak hunger, and then follow it by whatever you normally eat. Not only will you guarantee that you have room for your produce intake, but this will naturally fill you up and cause you to eat less of the Fake Food. This doesn't always work, but it is effective most of the time, which is going to help later on.

- Know your serving sizes. When you reach the point where you are eating eight servings a day, you'll find that the rest of the food you eat will be cut down by nature of being full from the produce. Here is a little guide for some common vegetables so you can eyeball how many servings you ate through the day. [1]

- ½ cup cooked green or orange vegetables (for example, broccoli, spinach, carrots or pumpkin)

- ½ cup cooked dried or canned beans, peas or lentils

- 1 cup green leafy or raw salad vegetables

- ½ cup sweet corn

- ½ medium potato

- 1 medium tomato

- 1 medium apple, banana, orange or pear

- 2 small apricots, kiwi fruits or plums

- 1 cup diced fruit

- As we talk about later in this book, affirmations have a weird way of changing our thought process. Try using them to help you enjoy eating new foods quicker than by trial alone. Let's say you have always believed yourself to hate brussels sprouts but found a new recipe you're going to try using the dreaded sprouts. While you are cooking them up, repeat in your head (or out loud if you don't mind your family looking at you strange), "I love brussels sprouts! I absolutely adore brussels sprouts more than I love chocolate! If it was my dying day, and I had one meal left, it would be nothing but brussels, brussels and more brussels! They are my favorite food!" While this will feel strange, try to really get into it and believe it with every ounce you can muster. You will be surprised at how quickly these beliefs start to cement themselves into your mind. It may not be the first few times, but eventually, you will actually believe brussels sprouts to be the end all, be all when it comes to veg. Sounds crazy, I know, but it works.

- As said above, experiment with different flavors. Use soy sauce, butter, oils, salt, pepper, herbs and spices with abandon. Go for a rich side dish using cheese, butter, tahini, or peanut butter. If you like Mexican food, make or buy a great spice blend and rub onto your veggies before roasting. Same goes for Indian, Thai, or any type of food you may be craving.

- Try to pick lots of colored vegetables to mix together. The brain craves nutrients from different sources and loves seeing a plate of rainbow-colored vegetables. It will stimulate a part of the psyche that may have been laying dormant for years. Try to make your plate look as gorgeous as possible, so when you sit down you actually feel like you are having a fancy meal.

Eating this way, will not only build your Happy Buzz, but it will do so without any extra effort on your part. It will start pushing out the urge to eat the processed junk food you are used to bingeing on. Fruits and vegetables are not only loaded with vitamins and nutrients that will give you loads of energy, but they will fill your stomach up and help you naturally fight those ravenous cravings for a quick fix

<u>STEP 2 :</u>

Protein Power

←————\\————→

Now that we are eating a good mix of greens every day, we will add in another essential nutrient to achieve our Happy Buzz: Protein. We've all heard about bodybuilders drinking raw eggs, and slamming protein shakes all day to get their huge muscles. If your goal is to get all oiled up and bust some moves on a stage, then go hogs wild and eat protein all day, every day. For the rest of us, we want to start adding in good proteins at every meal because protein gives your body a kick in the pants and enables you to undertake more physical activity with ease. Yes, protein helps build muscles, but that doesn't mean you will be walking around like the hulk just because you eat a lot of it. Eating protein makes the muscles you already have, stronger, more firm and better able to function. In turn, this speeds up your metabolism (the process that helps your body turn food into energy), which in turn, gives you more energy and quicker. Where fruits and veg gives your body immediate hits of energy, protein gives it the fuel that will burn for a long time. Both are essential for the Happy Buzz.

There is a lot of debate on what type of protein is best. Should we drink protein shakes? Is red meat good or bad? Can we eat eggs, and if so, how many? Where does Dairy fit into the picture? What about the protein from carbohydrates, should we avoid or eat?

You probably already know the answer since you have made it this far into the book, but I'll tell you again. If it is not processed, if it has one ingredient, and if it makes you feel better after you eat, then go nuts! Speaking of nuts, they are a great source of protein, so add them into your daily meal plan. However, when we are dealing with protein, there are a few caveats we need to keep in mind when planning out our meals. This is a category of food that different people can have different reactions to, so I'm going to show you how to determine if you have sensitivities to certain proteins. None of these foods are "bad," but they might not optimize your energy levels like we would like, so we need to figure out how to choose what suits us best.

Let's look at cheese to show how we determine what kind of protein helps build our buzz. There are many, many foods that taste better with cheese. Everything from a pound of mozzarella spread over roasted eggplants, soaked in an herby tomato sauce, to eating a slice straight from the fridge to using cheese as one would a seasoning. One person might be able to grate parmesan cheese over their roasted vegetables, sprinkle some feta into their salad and have a little mozzarella with a piece of fruit, and not have any issues. That same person might decide to make a queso dip later that evening and immediately have heartburn and bowel issues (you know what I'm talking about). Bowel issues and heartburn are not energy givers, those issues mean that something is not working smoothly in the body. This person should note that while a sprinkling of cheese can help them enjoy their vegetables more (energy giver), when they make cheese the main feature of their meal, it wreaks havoc on their body (energy sucker). So, this person can enjoy cheese, but only in moderation since their goal is to have as much energy as possible. Only you will be able to tell where your limit is for some of these items, but just use your body as your guide. If eating red meat, like a steak, makes you feel like you need to sit down or take a nap afterwards, then maybe try using red meat in a different way. Make a stir fry using only a few strips of beef as a flavour enhancer, rather than the main part of the meal. Test out different methods before throwing out an entire food group. The solution just may be to eat a much smaller amount than you normally would. If your body still feels sluggish after a small amount, it's probably a good idea to avoid that food item. It's just not worth feeling crappy all day, just to have a few minutes of eating a tasty food. Substitute another item that gives you the Happy Buzz and you'll enjoy life a lot more.

Surprisingly, there are quite a few grains and pulses that also pack a big punch in terms of protein. Oats are consistently on nutritionist's lists of super foods for being high in protein (along with fiber, potassium, and iron). However, for me, oats don't give me a big energy hit, they leave me neutral or worse, tired. So, instead of avoiding them altogether, I eat oatmeal a few times a week, but instead of having it for breakfast, I eat it as my last meal of the day. It helps me sleep better and avoid the headaches and body aches that come with eating other refined carbohydrates like bread to help me sleep. So, keep in mind that while all these foods are good sources of protein, you really need to determine when to eat them during your day, how much is too much, and for some, you might want to avoid altogether if they don't make you feel well afterwards. Your judgement is better than anybody else's.

The next page consists of a chart of common food items and the amount of protein each contains. As you can see, animal proteins are much higher than their plant-based counterparts. As usual, it's hard to get a definitive number for the amount of protein to eat each day. Different diet plans, nutritionists, and doctors all recommend different amounts depending on their food plan. Refer to your doctor if you want more information. I aim for 50-60 grams of protein every day. With that amount, I don't feel like I'm overdoing meat, and I get a stable release of energy all day long. Tweak your numbers until your body feels optimized, but that number is a good place to start.

Below is a list of high protein foods that will help give your body that Happy Buzz.

Approximate measurements

Meat	Amount	Protein
Chicken	3 oz.	26g
Beef	3 oz.	20-25g
Pork	3 oz.	23g
Turkey	3 oz.	24g
Salmon	4 oz.	27g
Shrimp	4 oz.	26g
Eggs	1 egg	6g
Beans	1 cup	16g
Quinoa	1 cup	8g
Peanut Butter	2 Tbsp.	7g
Nuts	¼ cup	40g
Milk	1 cup	8g
Yogurt	1 cup	25g
Cheese	2 slices	10g
Butter	1 Tbsp.	0.1g

Oatmeal	½ cup	7g
Spinach (raw)	1 cup	1g
Asparagus	1 cup	3g
Broccoli	1 cup	3g
Brussels Sprouts	1 cup	3g
Cauliflower	1 cup	2 g
Carrots	1 cup	1g
Lentils	1 cup	18g
Pumpkin Seeds	1 cup	12g
Chia Seeds	1 oz.	5g
Flaxseed	1 oz.	5g

Brain Hacks

The good news is this step is relatively easy for most people to implement. Most people have no problem identifying a couple of protein sources they really enjoy. When working on this step, be sure to pair your protein with a fruit or veg. This is a winning energy combo and will be sure to stabilize your Happy Buzz for hours. Since we have such an easy time with protein, this is a good opportunity to start making positive associations for your fruit and vegetables. Let's say you can't get excited about apples, but you love cheese. Well guess what? Apples and cheese go exceptionally well together, especially cheddar. So, start training your brain to associate the protein with your healthy produce. "Yes, it's time to eat a chunk of cheddar" will slowly turn into, "YES! It's time for apples and cheddar!" It will be the new peanut butter and jelly in your brain. They belong together. Speaking of peanut butter, that's another tasty protein that goes great with fruit and veg. Celery, carrots, and pears, oh my. Positive associations in the brain, make it easier to form new habits. So, look for as many new pairings as you can find.

As always, make sure to note your elevated energy levels after each meal or snack, to reinforce to your brain that eating this way makes you feel good.

Tips and Tricks

When it comes to protein, the best trick is to be prepared. When cooking meat, prepare a little extra and set aside for a later snack or new dish. Also, there is no shame in eating the same thing every day. If you really like celery sticks with peanut butter as an afternoon snack, then eat that as your afternoon snack every day. Variety is indeed the spice of life, but monotony may help you spice up your own life as you move toward a healthy diet.

Below are a few quick and easy ideas for a quick boost of Produce Protein.

- Cheddar cheese and apples

- Feta cheese and roasted peppers

- Mozzarella and Tomatoes

- Chicken and broccoli

- Smoked Salmon, Cream cheese, and capers

- Shrimp Ceviche

- Omelette

- Peanut butter and strawberries

- Handful of nuts and a peach

- Oatmeal with sliced banana

- Lettuce wrap with leftover meat

- Chia seeds, Yogurt and fresh fruit

- Cream and cherries with pumpkin seeds sprinkled on top

- Hard boiled eggs soaked in soy sauce over arugula

- Hummus with carrots and peppers

- Biltong and an orange

- Omelette with salsa

- Tuna salad in an avocado bowl

After you have developed the habit of incorporating the right amount of **Produce + Protein** into your diet, you should be feeling pretty good. Your body is starting to heal, and all the nutrients you are ingesting are going to start levelling out and be a constant, instead of hit and miss. Take this positive state of mind as we begin the next step, you will need it, because the next step can be brutal.

STEP 3:

No More Junk in the Trunk

So, at this point you should be feeling a change in your energy levels. You're eating 6-8 servings of produce a day and eating protein with each meal. Not only should you be feeling the immediate effect that these nutritious foods have on your body, but the habit of eating this way should start to be taking hold. You're doing a great job and should be really proud of yourself for completing the first two steps. You are already eating healthier than most humans, and with this next step we are going to take our energy into turbo drive.

Up to this point, we've only focused on adding food into our diet. This next step is the first time we are going to cut something out. The reason we do this step third, is because by adding fresh produce and proteins, you've probably already started doing step three without even thinking about it.

Step Three: Cutting out Fake Food (processed foods, refined carbohydrates, and sugar).

We are going to keep it real here; this is the hardest step for most people. Processed foods, refined carbs, and sugar are all different names for the same product: cheap fake food filled with sugar, useless junk carbs, fat, high amounts of salt, and processed oils. These foods have been designed by food manufacturers to not only taste as good as possible, but also be highly addictive to the average human. Don't feel guilty if the processed food demon has a tight grip on your mind, body, and soul. These foods have become so commonplace in current society, that it feels almost impossible not to indulge ourselves. The big food giants know we are on to them, so they have come out with new types of fake food, but this time they have packaged it up, with nice "feel-good" words like, high in fiber/calcium/iron/etc. Low fat/sugar/carb/fun can be found plastered across everything from bagels to ice cream. All available to buy for a cheap price that is sure to appeal to the masses. There's just one problem.

None of this is food.

Sure, it looks like food, but looks can be deceiving. These foods are comprised of a few natural ingredients that have been processed so deeply that they don't even resemble their original form. Then they're mixed with chemicals and dyes to further cut down the amount of actual food and beef up the quantity. When other drug dealers do this, it's called lacing the drug, or cutting it, meaning they add in cheap and dangerous stuff to bulk out their stash. Food manufacturers do the same thing, but because we don't see these foods as drugs, we give them a pass. But make no mistake, the processed foods, refined carbohydrates, and sugar filled goods are just as addictive, and deadly, as the crap people buy in a dark alley. Instead of looking like a meth head, these drugs will make you overweight, lose your health, and suck the life out of you. Sure, eating a bag of chips every day for a week won't see you drop dead today, but eventually, they will kill you. Our most lethal diseases are caused by these foods. Heart attacks, strokes, diabetes, and various types of cancers have all been traced back to our overwhelming dependence on Fake Food. Literally. We must get off them. No cheating, no going back, we must kick the habit and say no to drugs.

Luckily, from our first two steps, we've already seen that we can push them out of our diet by adding in new foods. In this step, we are going to slowly transition from processed foods, to making our own versions at home if we really, desperately crave them (we'll call this the transition phase), and then once we have everything gone that comes in a cardboard box or a plastic wrapper, we will stop making the sugary food altogether.

Now, some of you reading this will feel like this is an impossible step. The lure is just too strong, you have a sweet tooth, you love baking, you need a cookie with your coffee or tea... The excuses are a mile long. Just put that to the side and put some faith in yourself. Follow the steps, and you will get there. I promise. Not only will you get there, but you won't even crave those foods anymore. Looking at a package of cookies on the shelf won't phase you and you will actually prefer a nice tasty piece of fruit. Don't stress about it, and it probably won't take as long as you think. Everybody knows of a lifelong smoker who quit, a heavy drinker who is stone cold sober, or a formerly overweight individual who now does cross training and runs marathons for fun. These changes are possible, no matter how difficult you think the process will be. The people who have made these huge, positive changes in their lives all started in the same place. They had the same self-doubts. The same fears. Yet, the all took that same first step. They resolved to quit, and they did. You can do it too. Even if you don't believe in yourself, just put one foot in front of the other, and we will get through this part as painlessly as possible.

Why are processed foods so addictive?

Have you ever thought about what time of day or what type of situation you're in when you really have those heavy sugar cravings?

Back when I used to eat sugar by the bucketful, I always had extreme cravings when I was tired. I'd wake up in the morning and want a few spoons of sugar, with a little coffee to make it go down smooth. Then cereal, or toast and jam. Maybe some orange juice. It's our bodies way of getting a quick kick of energy when we need it. The problem with this, is that while we do get a burst of energy from the sugar, we also get a crash right after. Leading us to need more sugar. The cycle continues all day until you can finally go back to bed. It's no wonder that sugar is known to give us a hit of the "feel good" hormone, dopamine. Getting a little hit of energy, *does* feel good. It makes us happy for a short period of time, because we feel a bit more revved up than usual. Keep in mind though, a junkie also feels good when they get their hit. The brain isn't always the best gauge of what 47ehaviour is good for us or not.

Another interesting fact about sugar is that it's known to mess with your body's censors. We all have little pathways from our gut to our brain that relay information and inform our actions. If we eat a steak and a salad, our gut sends a signal to our brain that we are full, and to stop eating. It is difficult to overeat and be overweight when eating a whole foods diet. Whole food sends the signal to your brain, and if you try to keep eating anyways, the signal strength increases. Thanksgiving is a holiday, where we all consciously eat until our collective brain signals are screaming at us to unbuckle our pants and put the fork down. We all sit around in a food coma for a few hours afterwards, while our poor brain is trying to figure out, what just happened and wondering why we didn't heed it's warning. After your food starts digesting, the brain realizes we have stopped our binge and starts to let you feel a bit normal again. Now, let's say we take the turkey, potatoes, green beans, yams and added up all the calories and realize we ate 3,000 calories at our Thanksgiving meal. Well, we start to see why our brain is sending us the message that we are full and done. That's all the calories we need for the day (and then some), and your brain is working properly by telling you that you've achieved your food intake for the day.

The next day is Black Friday, and you decide to go out and get some bargains at the shops. After pushing your way through the mobs to get that TV for 50% off, your brain signals to you that you're hungry and need to eat. You're out, so you stop into a fast food joint. You grab a double cheeseburger, some fries, and a milkshake to enjoy. You eat it and don't feel hungry anymore. You get up and head over to the next mosh pit battle for those kitschy toaster ovens or hot new electronic device. Without realizing it, you just ate another 3,000 calorie meal. Same as the day before. The difference is that yesterday you were in pain from eating too much; today you aren't bothered at all. Why is this?

Well, on Thanksgiving we tend to have a lot of old fashioned, real food. The pathway between gut and brain works well when we eat real food. After stuffing our face with turkey, potatoes, and green bean casserole, our brain is easily able to send out the message that we have had enough. Our brain understands what we have consumed, knows where to send it, and has a system set up to let our other body parts know how to digest the different elements of our meal. On Black Friday we ate the same amount in calories, but we ate fake food. Guess what? Our gut to brain pathway tried to process the fake food in the same way as the real food and there was a glitch. The brain couldn't read the message from the gut, and everything got lost in translation. Our brain sees some proteins, fat, and carbs, but they aren't really the same as the Real Food that our brain has evolved to process. So, the brain goes about trying to figure out how much we ate, tries to alert our other organs and cells that there is some sort of food that needs to be digested, or nutrients that need to be sent out through the body, but it's all a bit hazy. The Fake Food looks like something it can make use of, but our brain just isn't completely sure how to handle it. Our brain never ends up figuring out what is going on and doesn't send us the message that we are full. Sugar/processed foods are known to inhibit the receptors in the brain. When you eat the fake food, you're making it very difficult on your brain (and yourself) to ever feel full. Imagine your body as a car that takes diesel.

If you put in regular gasoline by mistake, you are going to have some serious issues and need to take your car to a mechanic. While gasoline and diesel seem similar to us, cars engines (their brains) are only designed to use one or the other. If you put in the wrong fuel, the engine doesn't know what to do with it, and will try to make it work, but ultimately, it's going to wreck your wheels.

When we switch to a whole food diet, we allow our gut-to-brain path to operate properly, and in turn, we start receiving the messages again. It's so much easier to eat healthy, and know how much, and when, to eat, when your message center is working. Not only that, but when we eat whole foods, our body's cycle will fall back into its proper rhythm. Our gut tells the brain we are empty, the brain gives out the hunger message, we put food into the gut, the gut tells the brain it's full, and the brain tells us to stop. Then the brain CC's the digestive system that we have a full gut, old Mr. Colon puts his hard hat on and gets to work.

Sugar is the Devil

Americans eat, on average, around three_pounds of sugar each WEEK! You know those medium sacks of sugar at the store? That's a pound. We are eating three of those Every. Single. Week. That's just the average, some of us are eating even more. Sugar is added to every packaged food item these days. From all types of bread, to pasta, to yogurts, fast food burgers and fries and even into "healthy" items like protein bars and low-fat options. It's everywhere. We discussed above how fake food products damage the gut-to-brain message center, but we really need to look at just how bad sugar is for the body. Not only does sugar cause the brain to be unable to tell when you are full, thus making you overeat, but sugar is known to suck the energy out of your body. Some people feel as if they are constantly existing in a brain fog, feeling as though they are constantly struggling to remember things, stay on task, and keep track of the day. Constant, high levels of sugar, cause fluctuations in your blood sugar. These fluctuations affect not only the gut-to-brain path, but ALL the paths in your brain. The sugar depletes certain hormones we need, it causes misfiring left, right, and center. It can get so bad, that your insulin system essentially quits working for you. This is the path to Type 2 Diabetes.

It is essential that in our next step, we get rid of sugars, and all the foods that contain them (meaning all processed foods), once and for all. It takes a couple of weeks to get over the hard part of the cravings. However, unlike some other diets, we are allowed to eat healthy fruits in our eating plan. Just make sure it's paired with a protein. There are two ways of doing this process; Cold Turkey, or the Phase Out. Just as with smoking, some people do better just quitting all at once and suffering a short period of time, while others need to vape, or wear a nicotine patch. It doesn't really matter, as long as you are moving in the right direction. If you quit cold turkey, it will be a few weeks of feeling cranky, and uncomfortable. If you choose to do a slow phase out, you will still have moments of crankiness and irritability, but it might not be as severe. Below are two guides to help you get through this step depending on what plan you decide to take.

Cold Turkey

This is exactly how it sounds, you quit the fake foods all at once. Cold turkey is the preferred method of quitting. Just like ripping a band-aid off, deciding to end the sugar addiction, and toughing through the uncomfortable urges. The best way to do this it to set aside some time on the day you decide to quit. Go through your kitchen and your home with a trash bag and gather up all processed food. All sugar. All flour. All premade bread. If your food came in a cardboard box or a plastic bag with a brand on it, you can toss it. Once you have everything gathered, throw it away (or donate to a food shelter if you'd like). After saying goodbye to this toxic junk, go to the grocery store. Fill your cart with all the new Produce + Protein you've been adding to your diet. Get some nice high fat treats you might have always felt were off limits on diets. Some high-quality cheese or a lovely marbled steak. Grab a few pints of berries, and cream to dip them into. Salty nuts are a great sugar craving fix. When you get home, wash and put away all your Real Food so that it looks beautiful and is easy to eat when needed. Put a big bowl of fruit and vegetables out on the counter for snacks. Then just get through the next couple of weeks. The hardest part will be first 24-48 hours. After that, the cravings will subside to manageable levels. It will still take another few weeks to really kick the habit and get to the place where you aren't craving sugar at all. Even then, you may have a moment here and there, but overall, it will be relatively easy after that point. When you think of how much energy you will have, and how many diseases whose risks will be substantially lowered, a couple of weeks of annoyance is well worth it.

Transition Method

If you really can't imagine yourself able to quit the Fake Food cold turkey, then set up a plan to wean yourself off the junk. Think of this method as a "sugar patch." Smokers get to utilize a bevy of quitting aids, but for those battling Fake Food addictions, they just have to tough it out. It's okay if you need a quitting aid, but since you are still going to be dabbling with the very thing you are trying to quit, you need to be extremely vigilant and strict about the amount of Fake Food you are eating. It's a good idea to download a calorie counting app to be able to log your food. As time goes by, you want the grams of sugar you are eating to go down. That's a good guide to knowing you are eating better. As long as it is moving in that direction, you are on the right path. If your sugar consumption is going up, or staying the same, then that is your signal that something is going wrong, and you need to make some changes.

So, when we use the transition method, we start the same way as going cold turkey. Go through your kitchen with a trash bag and throw out (or donate) all the Fake Food. (***you already said this on page 32) Then decide on one or two Fake Foods for the week that you will allow yourself to enjoy. This can be anything from bread to a piece of chocolate. The only condition is that it must be a small portion, meant to take the edge off, not to eat as much as you want. So, let's say you picked bread and chocolate. The first day, go as long as you can without it, focusing on your meals consisting of Produce + Protein. When the cravings get too strong, allow yourself the small portion of fake food to take the edge off. The next week, we use the same method, but this time with only one portion of Fake Food per day. Try to go as long as possible without eating the Fake Food, by using tasty Real Food to fill up on instead. Make sure to eat your Produce + Protein so that you don't get too hungry. Hunger is a huge trigger for sugar cravings, so keep hunger at bay during this time. Cheese and nuts are great Real Foods that fill up the stomach, and still feel indulgent. Eat them as you need to get through this process. The following week do not have any Fake Food in the house. Try to kick the habit at this point. You have taken your sugar intake down to low levels, so you will be able to use willpower at this time. Just stick with it, knowing that the first 24-48 hours is the worse, and after that, you only have a few weeks of discomfort left. After that, it will all be over.

Natural Sweeteners

You may be wondering about so called, natural sweeteners. Honey, Maple Syrup, Agave Syrup, Coconut Sugar, etc., can all be considered "Real Food." While this is true, sugar is sugar. Earlier in the book, I said that once we quit Fake Food, we will be able to fine tune our diets to find the foods that really make us feel energized, and cut the food that might act as a sleeping aid. Natural sweeteners are no exception to the rule. Sugar is sugar. While natural sweeteners may have a few more nutrients than ordinary table sugar, they are still sugar and will take your body on the rollercoaster of the sugar rush. Once you have completely quit Fake Food, a little here and there may be fine for some, but if you find yourself craving more and more, stop and realize that eating them will only lead you back to a lethargic life. The overwhelming majority of people can't regulate their sugar intake, and there is no reason to think that you are one of the lucky ones. It's best to avoid all sweeteners and get your sugar rush from fruit alone. Trust me, once you are off the Fake Food, your tastes will change and you won't need the constant sugar fix that is plaguing you now. Once you have quit the Fake Food, a few berries will suffice any cravings for dessert. Eating natural sweeteners will just delay your progress, so even though they are Real Food, for all intents and purposes, think of them as Fake.

A Note on Cheat Days

A lot of diets advocate "cheat days" to entice people to follow their diet plan. Since this isn't a "diet" we need to be honest about "cheat days." We are eating for sustained, and stable energy levels. Having a day of the week where we go out and eat a bunch of Fake Food will not allow us to achieve the Happy Buzz. Every time you "cheat" and go back to eating Fake Food, you have just created two big problems for yourself. One, you now have to spend a few days allowing your body to process the Fake Food, clear the junk out of its system, and get back into it's normal mode of functioning. This means, less than stellar energy output. If you do this once a week, then you are only really getting the full effect of eating for energy for about half the week. In our new way of thinking, we know that this isn't the goal, we want ourselves to feel great all the time.

Secondly, we have now experienced that the Fake Food addiction is real. We have experienced the cravings, the withdrawal symptoms, the struggle to get through the process. Here's the bad news, just like any other addiction, when we relapse, there's a very high chance that we have to start the entire process over again. When a drug addict quits, we know they went through hell to come off the drugs. If they came back and said, they quit, but they are going to use one time per week, we would know that they didn't really quit, but that it was just a matter of time before they were back on drugs full time. Fake Food addiction is not a joke, and there is no such thing as dabbling in it as an ex-addict. Every time we relapse, there's a high chance that we will be right back in the throes of addiction and will have to start back at the beginning. Treat Fake Food as you would any other addictive substance, and once you have gotten over the addiction, stay far away from the stuff. Don't tempt yourself, don't dabble in it— just steer clear.

***

No matter what method you choose to kick the Fake Food addiction, once this step is completed, things get a lot easier. Your energy levels will stabilize quickly and you will be able to get off the sugar high roller coaster. At this point, you are ready to lose any of the extra weight you don't need, and you are ready to really start tweaking your diet for optimal energy, optimal feel good habits, and optimal happiness. Congratulations, you have come out the other side of an extremely difficult addiction. You deserve to feel proud of yourself, and you should.

STEP 4:

Get Moving, Preferably Outdoors

"One helpful trick to keep yourself from getting burned out may actually be as simple as taking a short walk in nature, according to _a study by the University of Michigan._

The study, published in _Frontiers in Psychology_, suggests that taking 20 minutes to stroll in nature can reduce your stress hormone levels. The study coined this remedy as a "nature pill."

The study rounded up participants, asking them to take a walk for 10 minutes or more, at least 3 times a week. Levels of the stress hormone cortisol were measured using saliva swabs both before and after the so-called "nature pill." The _study found_ that after the walks cortisol was cut by 10 percent on average."

-Andrea Romano, Travel and Leisure Magazine

When those of us who don't exercise _think_ of exercise, we probably have visions of sweaty bodies bouncing around on contraptions in the gym, typically accompanied by crappy music blasting at insane levels, and ridiculously muscled figures posing in front of the weights. The gym has become a symbol of health and pro-active behavior in today's society. We spend big bucks to belong to these fitness centers in the hope that we will develop a habit and get super ripped and healthy. However, as a lot of us know, what actually happens is that few people manage to incorporate the gym into their regular schedule. The majority of us use our membership as a way to feel guilty every month. Not only do we get to watch the money drain out of our accounts, we get the added bonus of having a reminder to berate ourselves for not following through on our exercise plans. Failure on all counts.

A well-used gym membership can be a great investment in your health when it is used regularly. Otherwise, it falls into the category of demotivating. When we are executing The Energy Diet, we try to avoid things that demotivate us. Exercise doesn't have to be all pain, for the gain. Our bodies are designed to move, they're made for walking and running long distances, primed for standing upright for long periods of time, engineered to be out hunting or gathering food. Your body wants to move. It wants to be out in the world, exploring and taking in fresh air while the sun is shining down on your face, or even when the rain is pouring down on your head. Your body is able to walk through rain, snow and slush and survive. You can go outside at any time of the year, and your body will acclimate and still work in the way it's intended. Use this instinct to your advantage and get outdoors for a major energy boost every day. Walking in nature, whether that's a forest, along a dusty trail, or even through a beautiful park in the city, will take your stress down, and boost your Happy Buzz.

Enjoying the great outdoors has more health benefits than just getting your exercise minutes completed for free. When you walk, or run, or bike outdoors rather than the gym you also:

- Increase energy levels.

- Feel as if you are in a good mood.

- Lower stress.

- Help clear your head.

- Reduce the risk of heart disease.

- Increase your metabolism.

- Burn more calories due to the terrain.

- Decrease cholesterol.

- Reduce blood pressure.

- Improve your breathing.

- Decrease resting heart rate.

- Help fight depression and anxiety.

- Improve Optimism.

Once you start the habit of spending time outdoors every day, you will notice that it becomes an addiction of its own. Your brain and energy levels will enjoy it so much, that on the days when you just aren't able to make it for your walk, you will miss it. What a great thing to get hooked on. Moving out in the fresh air is so intrinsic to human nature, that when you start allowing yourself to get out, your animal instincts will take over and you will be surprised at the reaction from your mind and body. Have you ever seen those cat videos on YouTube where the owner places a cucumber next to the cat and the poor cat notices it and jumps across the room? Apparently, the cat believes it to be a snake and knows it needs to move—quickly. Now, these cats are usually house cats that have never been outside, never seen a snake, never been in a threatening situation from a predator. Yet, their bodies instantly react to this stimulus in an immediate way. Nobody quite understands how this fear gets passed on through the generations of cats, but some theorize that it is imprinted into a cat's mind, and their body knows how to react, even in unfamiliar situations. Humans seem to have similar imprints, and once we recognize those, we can use them to our advantage. Walking outdoors might bring up connections to when humans were hunters and gatherers. For millions of years, we spent all day outdoors, walking through nature. Maybe when we get out there, something clicks and makes us feel as if we are back to doing what we are meant to be doing, biologically. Maybe that's the reason that walking through a forest is so much more energizing and calming than walking on a treadmill.

Whatever the reason, take advantage of all the extra benefits of getting physical while outside. There's no doubt that adding this activity will bring massive enjoyment to your life for a multitude of reasons. All you need to do is find a beautiful spot, put your shoes on and go.

STEP 5:

Getting your Zzzzzzzzs

This step is a no-brainer. Getting a good night's sleep is essential for having maximum energy. You can get everything else right, but if you are consistently engaged in a sleep deficit, you won't be able to acheive the Happy Buzz. Sleep needs vary between adults, but most adults need between 7-9 hours of sleep per day. While it would be nice to be able to just sleep whenever we feet tired. Unfortunately, most of us have to adhere to a schedule and are blocked from taking a nap when we fancy. The boss doesn't appreciate finding us snoozing after lunch when we are being paid to work. Likewise, we typically have a time in the morning we must be up by, whether for kids, or school, or work. So, we must schedule in our sleep time to make sure we get the right amount.

Sleep is a strange topic today; you will consistently hear people bragging about their unhealthy habits. "Oh, I was out at that new bar all night, only got a couple hours of sleep last night, but here I am." Or, "I binge-watched this show on Netflix and next thing I knew, it was two in the morning." I always feel like asking, why are you telling people this? You wouldn't go around telling everybody that you ate an entire cake the night before and expect that to be a conversation starter. Nobody would be impressed; they would probably look at you with immense pity. We need to start valuing our sleep schedules. I guard my own sleep in the same way I guard my children's sleep. If we are invited out and it's past bedtime, we will pass on the activity. Exceptions are very rare, because I know that if enough sleep isn't had, everybody will have a tough next day; if not few days. It's just not worth it.

We know that sleep deprivation makes us tired the next day, but there are long term effects of not getting enough shut eye. When we sleep our body goes into recuperation mode. During our down time, our body heals its damaged cells, the immune system gets a boost, and your cardiovascular system recharges. Besides the health benefits for your body, your brain gets nurtured, allowing your gut-to-brain message center to work at peak performance, along with other recovery. Recent neurology findings theorize that sleep gives your brain the time to remove toxins that build up during the day. During sleep, there is an increase of brain fluid that seems to act as a dishwasher, clearing out the build-up. Neurologists are trying to find the connection between sleep disorders and brain diseases like Alzheimer after finding many correlations. Sleep is very important, and we need to take it seriously. Depending on what time you wake up in the morning, will determine your bedtime. If you get up at 6am, this means you should be *asleep* by 10pm; and notice the word asleep was used instead of "going to bed." If it takes a while to fall asleep, then bedtime needs to be pushed up to an earlier time.

So, we have two issues that we need to overcome in order to ensure we are getting enough sleep. First, we need to schedule our days, so that we don't run out of time and end up staying awake longer than intended. The easiest way to do this is to set up a bedtime and go to bed at the same time every night. Some people like to stay up late on the weekends and have a sleep-in the next morning. While it's understandable to take advantage of your days off from work, sleep experts agree that a set sleep schedule is necessary. That means that even if you want to stay up all night on Saturday evening, if you want to make sure you are optimized, you'll want to go to sleep the same as you would on a Monday night, and wake up the next morning at the same time you'd get up during the weekday. Changing your bedtime every day can also lead to having a sleep disorder later down the line, so make a schedule and stick to it.

The second issue that people have is difficulty falling or staying asleep. There are too many types of sleep disorders to cover in this book, but if you try all the tricks and still can't get a good night's sleep, it's a good idea to see a doctor and see if anything serious is going on. Below we will talk about a few ideas to make your sleep time easy and refreshing, but if you have a genuine health issue, you will need medical intervention. However, most people are just approaching sleep in the wrong way, and with a few tweaks, can turn their sleep habits around. When we go to bed, we want to be tired from the day, get into bed, and fall asleep in a few minutes. Then we want to stay asleep until we are naturally awakened in the morning. If you get your sleep right, you will soon be able to ditch the alarm clock and be able to wake up in the morning feeling refreshed and full of energy. Sleep is a vast subject that fills entire books with directions on how to sleep, so once you get the general idea of how to sleep well, it's always worth doing extended research if you wake up and still are not feeling fully recharged.

How to Sleep

- A cold room will help you sleep. We've all been in the situation of trying to sleep on a hot and sticky night. It's almost unbearable. The sheets are damp and sticking to you, it's hard to breathe, and you end up tossing and turning the entire night. Conversely, a cold bedroom with a cozy bed helps get people in the mood to fall asleep. Now, if you live in a warm climate, it could be hard to maintain a cool room, but there are a few things you can do if you aren't able to run the air conditioner all night. Blackout shades for your window will block the sun from heating the room during the day, and also can help keep the room dark from outside light. There are also mattress and pillow covers that keep the bed itself cool. You can find them online by searching for cooling pad, cooling gel pad, etc. Look for a brand with great reviews and make the investment.

- No television in the bedroom. A lot of people like to watch their favorite shows while trying to nod off. This is a bad idea. You want your bedroom to be a place for two things, sleep and sex. That's it. Making your bed into a DeFacto couch makes it hard for your brain to know when the time comes for sleep. You want a clear connection in your mind between being in bed and sleeping. When you get into bed, you want your bed to associate that action with the sleep signal. Just like when you smell dinner cooking, your brain associates the aroma with a hunger signal, laying down in bed should have the same effect on our brain.

- Electronics should not be brought into bed. Looking at phones while trying to fall asleep has become a worldwide bad habit. Phones emit a certain a light of a wavelength called "blue light." This light is beneficial during the day, it heightens attention, quickens reaction times and helps with mood, but it's terrible at night. At night, we are evolved to want low light, basically the light emitted from a fire is about all we should be looking at. Now that we have electricity, our homes are lit up from the ceiling, floor lamps, table lamps, the television, our phones and tablets, and it's all transmitting light directly into our brains, making our brains think that it's daytime, and not bedtime. It's unreasonable to think we are going to sit around in a dark home all evening, so we have to think of ways to minimize our exposure. The best way to do this, is to configure your living space to have very dim light options. Buy low wattage or dimmable bulbs, use your fireplace, and turn electronics off an hour before bedtime. Reading a book in a dim room by the fire for an hour before bed, will put you in the sleep state a lot easier than being in a room with the television blaring at you, while staring at your phone without the blue light filter.

- Ignore the clock. When you are trying to fall asleep and are unable, it's easy to start stressing about how late it's becoming. Also, if you wake up in the middle of the night, looking at the clock can alert you from a foggy state. Set your alarm before you go to bed, turn your phone upside down to eliminate light, and leave it for the night. Looking at the clock and stressing about the time will not help you get more sleep. It will just add to your stress hormones and make it more difficult to settle.

If you still have trouble getting to sleep, you may suffer from a genuine sleep disorder, and seeking the help of a medical professional could be warranted. Some sleep disorders such as Sleep Apnea, or Restless Legs Syndrome need to be treated by a doctor, but these sleep tricks will still help once you get your disorder treated.

Optimization and Implementation

You Did It, Now What?

Congratulations, you have made it successfully through the steps. You have switched to a Real Food diet, getting outside more, and sleeping better. What to do now? Well, you could just leave it there. Simply doing these five steps has improved your life immensely. There is no doubt that you are feeling better than you have in a long time.

When you started reading this book, you might have skimmed through the chapters, looking for the gist of what you needed to do. Then you realized it was set up to go through step by step, in order to beat the addiction. So, you started the program, and slowly started making small shifts in your diet and behavior. You probably thought that you'd get to the other side and feel pretty good, but I'm guessing you weren't ready for the actual scope of how drastically your life has changed.

When we are stuck in the fog of Fake Food, are brain isn't functioning properly, our digestion is wonky, and we feel too tired to put much thought into anything extra. Once we come out of that fog though, it feels like we've stepped into a new world.

And we have.

Our old lifestyle seems so far away, and dreary. We now are starting to rediscover dormant desires and dreams we had shelved away, long ago. We have a new lease on life and are excited to start trying new things, revisit old hobbies, and participate in life in an entirely new way. It's hard to explain to others just how deep this change has become. It's in our soul, our very fundamentals have evolved in a short time.

One thing we might ask, is if there is more we can do. If these changes made such a huge impact, can we go even further? Now that we aren't suffering from a Fake Food addiction, we can appreciate the feelings that Real Food delivers. Maybe a banana in the morning is just the right burst of energy to get out the door. Maybe that banana is too sweet and leads to a slump in the morning. You are primed to start recognizing the nuance in Real Foods. For example, while I don't think there is anything inherently wrong with potatoes, I choose to not eat them. Why? Well, because they make me feel like a nap afterwards. I don't know if it's the carb count, or maybe it's because I associate potatoes with big meals, and sleepy afternoons. Regardless of the reason, they just sit in my stomach, and I don't feel energized after eating them. Likewise, if I eat eggs, I eat them in the evening. They don't make me sleepy, but they just don't sit great with me if I eat them after my walk in the morning. Instead, a salad and a cup of coffee gets me feeling great, and ready to go. That's what I usually eat for my first meal. My daughter, on the other hand, only wants eggs in the morning. She eats a few scrambled eggs with some avocado, and you can physically see her come from a droopy head and half asleep, to awake and perky and ready for the day. Everybody is a little different. Now that we've conquered the beast, we can really start fine tuning our diets to know what makes us feel best at different times of the day.

Part II of this book goes into some more interesting ways to fine tune our diet and activities for even more energy. Each chapter details new tricks to try, whether it is psychological, physical, or both. Feel free to skip around to what interests you and try combining different elements for the best results.

Hacking the Brain

- When we first start making changes in our life, the mind has a funny way of working against us. No matter how convinced you are of the changes a healthy diet can make in your life, you are also having some other, less helpful thoughts.

- "I won't be able to make the change permanent, so why bother?"

- "I can't cook, how am I meant to prepare all these meals everyday?"

- "I know sugar is terrible, but there's no way I can give it up."

- "Not only sugar, but also breads and pasta? This lady can shove it up her..."

- "My kids will never eat vegetables."

- "My kids will never give up their sweets and chips."

- "It's so much easier to grab a bag of chips for a snack, rather than try to prepare fruits and vegetables."

- "This is too much work, and I'm already exhausted."

- "I'm going to end up cooking multiple dinners to please everyone. Not worth it."

- "The last thing I want to do when I get home from work is cook a full meal."

- "I don't like vegetables."

- "I don't like fruit."

- "I need sugar in my coffee or tea in the morning."

- "What am I meant to feed myself/my family without all the basics?"

There's a good chance at least one of these thoughts have played through your mind while reading this book, and that's okay. In this chapter, we are going to learn some clever little tricks to help "hack" your brain. Hacking your brain is as simple as understanding why your brain behaves in certain ways, and then thinking up clever little tricks to outsmart it. Yes, in this discussion we will discuss the brain as a separate entity. While reading, think of your brain as a character separate from yourself, one that you can manipulate to your will if you just ask correctly. This makes it easier to emotionally detach from your own negative thoughts and start the process to overcome your own thinking and be able to enact these new healthy habits.

Brain Hacks

Affirmations

You've probably heard of affirmations before. Think of Stuart Smalley, played by Al Franken from that old SNL skit. Stuart stands in front of the mirror and says a series of corny lines to himself such as "I'm good enough, I'm smart enough, and doggone it, people like me." He goes through his lines whenever life gets him down. These clichés people speak to themselves are called affirmations. They are just a way to speak to yourself in positive sentences to counteract negative thoughts.

Now, this probably seems pretty corny to most, but if you read through any books or listen to interviews by successful people, you'll start to notice that many of those who have achieved their goals have used this method along the way. Why is that? Well, let's think about how our brain works. Don't worry this won't get too deep. Think of your brain as a map, there are billions of little roads in this map called Neurons. Now, when we think of roads, let's think of the different types of roads. We have big mega-highways that are well paved, well lit, straight, and to the point. You hardly notice driving on these roads because you can just sit back and drive without having to think too much. Now think of a little country lane. It's a dirt road, there are potholes everywhere with lots of twists and turns. You must go slowly and take your time until you get more used to the terrain.

The roads in your brain are your thoughts. You have certain pathways that are so well developed and paved, that going from impulse to thought to action is automatic. The big mega highways of our brains are habits. We don't even have to think about it, because we've driven down this road so many times that our body just reacts. Habits are great, and make life a lot easier, until we develop a bad habit. That's when it gets tricky. When we develop bad habits, we do things we know we shouldn't, but our road is just so well paved, that we don't think there is another route. If we try to get off the highway and take a different way, we may end up on an old country lane. We have to go slower, it takes longer and it can be a more stressful experience. We need to be aware of every move. Our brains work in a similar way. Habits and certain thoughts are very easy for the brain to process, but once we start a new experience, or try to implement a new habit, you have ventured into uncharted territory and your brain doesn't have a clear pathway made yet. It's easy to see why our bodies resist going that way. Usually, we give up and get back on the highway, even if it's taking us to the wrong place. Think of your dietary habits and make a quick list of eating patterns that you know you shouldn't do, but you still seem to do them anyways.

Some examples:

- Not eating enough fruits and vegetables.

- Late night snacking on the couch.

- Eating too many sweets.

- Eating too much fast food.

- Buying the same items at the grocery store, instead of buying healthier options.

These are your mega highways. It's not your fault for behaving this way. It's so heavily ingrained in your brain that it's automatic and very hard to change.

Affirmations are the brain hacks that help you find a new way.

Let's go back to our highway, we know we are going the wrong way, we know we need to get off, but when we take the offramp, we are back on this old country lane. This is new territory for us. It makes us uncomfortable and nervous. We might feel a little scared since we don't know exactly what the journey will look like. This is completely normal. We just need to get to know this new road, the more we drive on it, the less stressful it will feel. The more we drive on it, the more we know what to expect around every bend. The more we drive on it, the smoother the dirt becomes, the road starts to even out, it starts to expand a little by little, by every new tread pushing the dirt out. After a while, this new road is easy-peasy to drive, and we get right to our destination. This new road eventually gets made into a highway because you're driving down it so often.

This all makes sense as an analogy, but let's get back to how this relates to our brains, and why I need to do silly affirmations every day. Okay.

So, our brains are a map of neurons, every thought we have goes down a "road" in the brain. Every time we have a thought, it navigates a pathway through your brain. The more we have the thought, the smoother the pathway gets, the easier it is to drive on, and it gets a bit bigger and more well defined. If we think about our thoughts, we probably have quite a few mega highway roads going through our brains. For a lot of us, these thoughts can be very negative. We might have told ourselves, we are ugly, we're too fat, we aren't determined enough, we can never succeed. We have thought these so many times, that we have created a mega highway of terrible thoughts in our brain. We don't even need to think about it anymore, passing a mirror will set off a load of terrible, self-defeating thoughts without even trying.

Affirmations are the secret weapon to start building new roads. When you first start saying them to yourself, it will feel uncomfortable. Your brain might get right back on the highway of thinking you are stupid. Thinking you are a failure. The key is to keep on anyways. Every time your thoughts get on that highway, you take a quick turn onto this new and uncomfortable road. Your brain says, "you'll never be thin." You say, "I love eating healthy and my body is getting better every day." Your brain says, "this will never work." You say, "this will definitely work, because I know eating well makes me feel better."

Any negative thoughts must be actively combatted by your counterargument of positivity. At first, this will be tiresome and awkward. But, after some time, these new roads will be so big and smooth, that the old country lane will have morphed into your mega highway. The old one will have become overgrown with foliage, split lanes, and eventually turn into a pile of rubble. You don't use that road anymore. It will eventually be swallowed back into the pit where it belongs.

Some affirmations that have helped me along the way:

- I hate cookies.

- This delicious salad makes me feel so energetic.

- I will feel so good about myself once I accomplish this boring task.

- I hate chips.

- Fast food is the spawn of the devil.

- I hate cake because it gives me wrinkles.

- Mornings are my favorite time of the day.

- I love to pick up legos all over the floor (this was a tough one).

- Boxed food tastes like vomit.

- Chopping produce is really relaxing.

- I love listening to a book while making dinner.

- I love a long walk in the morning.

- A walk puts me in a good mood.

As you can see, you can use this hack to overcome ANYTHING in your life that must be done, but that, right now, you don't find enjoyable. You will be amazed at how fast your attitude starts to change if you really set to work. Any task you don't enjoy, whether that is eating a certain vegetable, to making your bed, can be overcome by simply talking to yourself in terms that reinforce your behavior. In effect; you can change any bad habit by simply talking to yourself. Isn't that kind of amazing? And this works in any facet of life. So, why don't you go make a list of your most pointless mega highways, come up with your rebuttals and start building your new roads today? What do you have to lose?

Positive Pairings

An easy way to train your brain to like things you may not like is to pair that object or activity with something you really like. Let's say you love listening to podcasts, and you also want to incorporate more walks into your week but are having a hard time getting motivated. The easy way to get yourself out and moving, is by mentally pairing your podcast with your walks. Don't allow yourself to listen to that podcast at any other point in the week, unless you are on a walk. Make a rule for yourself and stick with it. After a few times of doing this, your brain will start associating going for a walk with finally getting to indulge in your pleasure. In this example, you not only get the positive reward of finally getting to listen to your show, you also will be getting natural endorphins from being outside, exercising, and being proud that you worked out for the day. That's a total power pack of motivation that will make it much easier tomorrow to get out and do the same. Fairly quickly, you will have developed a walking routine, and it won't even feel like a chore. It will become something you look forward to doing. You get a huge dose of happiness from multiple angles just by performing this task each day.

We can do the same with food. Perhaps you love peanut butter, and you're the type of person who just sticks a huge spoon in the jar and eats it in pure bliss. Now, at the same time, you are trying to eat more fruits and vegetables but having a hard time getting motivated. No problem. We are going to make a positive pairing again. Every spoonful of peanut butter you eat out of the jar has to be paired with a piece of fruit. So, you grab your spoon and scoop some up, go sit down and eat it, but you need to have an apple alongside that spoonful. What happens if you eat the peanut butter and apple and you want more peanut butter? Easy. Go get another scoop of peanut butter and this time grab some celery sticks to accompany it. You are now rewiring your brain to associate these two foods together. Soon, it will be second nature to grab a piece of fruit when you are craving peanut butter. Use this too your advantage to add more healthy options into your diet while still enjoying the food you love.

Negative Consequences

We want to try to stay positive in our journey to the Happy Buzz, but sometimes we are going to mess up. That's okay. The great thing about rewiring our brain to think about food in terms of our energy levels, instead of our waistline, is that our mess ups can easily be overcome. If you've been eating for energy for a little while, and you mess up and have a meal full of processed fake food, you are going to feel it. It will be obvious to you because you will feel tired and lethargic afterwards. You may feel moody or get irritated easily. It will become quite noticeable to you the change in your demeanor when you give your body Fake Food instead of Real Food. Instead of beating yourself up for it, take a few moments and let your mind really absorb the negative consequences from eating the junk. Reinforce in your mind that you are now having a crappy afternoon because you ate pizza and a soda for lunch. Think about how you feel tired as those refined carbs and sugar course through your system. Think about the sugar high and then the painful crash from the soda. Pay attention to how much you dislike that feeling and blame it entirely on your lunch. Next time you are thinking of eating pizza and soda for lunch, try to remember how zapped you felt afterwards, and ask yourself if it's really worth the trouble.

Make Space

Part of our plan to go from junk food-aholics to Real Food nuts is to add in the good stuff first, and then take out the bad stuff once we have created some healthy habits. When we start trying to cut down on the Fake Food, we want to make it as difficult as possible for us to get our hands on the food. Let's say your favorite Fake Food consists of cookies and chocolate milk. At first, you don't believe that yourself to possess the willpower to quit cold turkey. So, what you do is move the location of where you keep your Fake Food. Right now, you probably keep all your food in the kitchen. There's a good chance your kitchen is quite near to where you sit down and relax. There's also a good chance that when you sit down and relax, you want your cookies. With your current set up, whenever you have a craving, you only have to walk a few feet to have your craving satisfied. Now, what would happen if you move the location of the cookies to another part of your home? Preferably the place furthest from your munchie spot, maybe even outside or in a garage. In this scenario, when you sit down and relax and get your cookie craving, you cannot just walk a few feet and grab them. You have to walk upstairs, or put shoes on to go outside, or make some sort of effort. While, there's a good chance you might still get them anyway, there will be an annoyance factor built in that may help you resist the urge. Each time you crave cookies, your brain will register annoyance. That's a good start. Once your brain overcomes that annoyance and walking up the stairs and getting a ladder out to get the cookies, you can make even more space between you and the cookies. Now, if you have a craving, you need to go out to the store and buy a pack. You no longer allow yourself to buy a full-size pack—only a snack size. So, now, every time you want those cookies, you must go to the store and buy them. If all you can buy is a full-size pack, then you'll buy those and throw away what you don't eat. Your brain will start associating this annoyance with the cookies and we now have a negative association being hardwired with craving those cookies.

While you are physically setting up obstacles for yourself and the junk, you simultaneously will set up healthy substitutions that are very easy to get to. On your kitchen counter, place a big bowl overflowing with pretty fruit and jars of nuts. Stock the refrigerator with precut veggies, or premade meats, boiled eggs, or salads. If you sit on the couch at the end of the day, and the kitchen is nearby, make it easy to grab a healthy snack. When you crave a cookie (a sweet craving), focus on your options instead of mindless wandering. Decide, what you want to do. You can either grab an apple and throw in a dark chocolate square, and go back to what you were doing, or you must get yourself together and go out to the store to get your cookie fix. Really think about it before choosing. Usually, the apple will satisfy your sweet tooth without much fuss. Yet, if you just really can't cope, you still have the option of going to the store for that cookie, all the while, reaffirming to your brain that this craving is a major annoyance to you.

Kids Eat Free

Have you ever been to a child's birthday party? They all follow a similar format. The kids arrive, they play and run around for an hour or two and start to get hungry. So, food is brought out, usually pizza, or chicken nuggets, or some other child friendly fare. Then we sing "Happy Birthday," followed by some cake and ice cream, and we send them back out to play. About an hour after, everyone is in tears, tantrums are being thrown, and the epic meltdowns begin. As parents, we know this means the party is about to end. The hosts start handing out the goody bags as a signal that it's time for everyone to go home, and parents start to drag their crying children out to the car for the ride home and long night of manic mood swings ahead.

Let's break down what is really happening here. When you arrive at the party, the kids are all happy and ready to have a great time. For a couple of hours, they are all getting along and enjoying whatever activity is set up for them. This is all completely normal and healthy behavior. Then after really exerting quite a bit of energy from all that playing, they realize they are hungry. Their bodies need refueling after expending so much energy. But then, we, as the adults, do something incredibly stupid. We stuff them full of processed foods, sugars, and refined carbohydrates, i.e., Fake Food. For the first hour or so after they eat, we can see the manic energy start to manifest itself. They run off with renewed vigor, running extra fast, jumping twice as high. Then the kids start getting a little aggressive with each other. You will notice that close friends start to bicker and the kids start pushing and shoving. The volume gets dialed up, with screaming and cries of "ouch, she bit me," ringing through the air. It's like a crescendo building and building. Then, the first tears. One child got hurt and starts crying, followed by another child running over to whine about a grievance. Before you know it, the party has turned into a cacophony of tears, tantrums and moaning.

What we are witnessing is the effect of processed and sugary food on our kids. The Fake Food hits their blood stream, and a manic energy seems to possess them. It continues to build for about an hour as their bodies are fully absorbing all the cake and pizza, with the child becoming more hyper and less reasonable with each passing moment. All at once, they crash, and an epic meltdown commences. It's an epic mood swing, and kids are not great at hiding their emotions.

When we feed our kids Fake Food, we are not only making their life more difficult, we are also making our own lives more difficult. We expect children to sit still in class all day, navigate social relationships, and diligently tend to their duties at home, all of which are already big tasks for a developing mind, and we decide to make it extra difficult by serving them up big plates of hormonal mood swings every day.

We start off the morning with a big bowl of sugar—I mean cereal. Then we send them off to school and expect them to not react when the insulin is hitting their blood stream making them want to swing from the ceiling. If they give in to this urge, they are punished. Later, when they crash and want to put their heads on their desks or feel very emotional, we scold them if they give into those whims. Lunch time comes around, by which they are at the phase of the cycle known as hunger and exhaustion, and we give them a peanut butter and jelly sandwich on white bread with a cookie and some fruit, all swallowed down with a bottle of juice. This sugar filled lunch starts the cycle all over. Their entire day is now about navigating the nasty sugar cycle, instead of trying to focus on learning, growing and exploring the world. Let's look at an example of what a typical child might eat for the day and see what is going on.

Sample Menu for a Young Child #1

- Breakfast: 1 Cup of Cheerios, 1 Cup of skim milk, and a banana

- Lunch: Peanut Butter and Jelly Sandwich (2 Tbsp. Each) on sliced white bread, 12 carrot sticks, and a bag of chips.

- Snack: Cheese crackers and an apple

- Dinner: 1.5 Cups of Penne Pasta with 1 cup of marinara sauce, with a slice of garlic bread.

This doesn't seem too bad at first glance right? How much sugar do you think is in this day's worth of food? Notice that there are no cookies, no juice, no dessert. They would be eating a little fruit, a few vegetable servings. It can't be that bad, can it? If a child were to eat this in a day, they would have eaten 92 grams of sugar for the day. That translates to 0.46 cups of sugar for the day, almost half a cup of sugar! This menu doesn't even consider extra sources of sugars, like a juice with their meal, or a little piece of candy for a "treat." Let's say we add in a box of juice with lunch and dinner, and a small snack size chocolate bar, how much sugar is in this child's diet now? Now we have fed this child 126 grams of sugar in a day, 0.63 cups! If we multiply this by seven days a week, we would be giving about 4.5 cups of sugar per week. That comes out to around two pounds of sugar per week. Keep in mind that this doesn't take into consideration all the extra sweets and treats they may also consume. A couple of fast food meals during a busy week, a birthday party filled with cake and ice cream on the weekend. You get the idea. It adds up quickly.

This breakdown is not meant to make you feel guilty, but it should be alarming. We would never allow our kids to dip a spoon into the sugar bag and eat two pounds in a week. We would be pouring it down the drain before we let them eat it Yet, in our society, we not only allow children to eat like this, but it's actually encouraged by our dietary guidelines. If you look at the bottom row of the food pyramid released by the United States Food and Drug Administration, you will see nothing but Fake Food—highly processed, sugar filled, refined carbohydrates. If you look at that bottom row, it's a bunch of beige food. Breads, pasta, cereals, and potatoes. This is the base of the pyramid, and the largest percentage of the pyramid, meaning we are meant to eat most of our food from this category. However, when we start looking at food as Fake Food versus Real Food, we can quickly see that only the potatoes are Real Food. Everything else is processed Fake Food. When we change our diet from Fake Food to Real Food, the sugar problem goes away by itself. Let's look at another meal plan for a child, this time eating only Real Food.

Sample Menu for a Young Child #2

- Breakfast: Scrambled Eggs (2 Eggs) with milk, and a banana.

- Lunch: Peanut Butter with celery sticks, Cheese and Ham roll ups, blueberries, and mixed nuts.

- Snack: Cream cheese and cucumbers with shredded ham on top

- Dinner: Chicken Breast covered in marinara sauce with melted cheese, carrot noodles, side salad.

If a child ate this in a day, they would have eaten 12 grams of sugar. That translates to less than one tablespoon. Not only that, but all the sugar would come from fruits and vegetables, food that adds fiber along with many essential nutrients. Not only will this child not be spending their day on the frantic roller coaster of Mood Swing Central, but they will also be getting shots of energy at regular intervals throughout the day thanks to the produce + protein equation.

This all sounds good in theory, right? It's all well and good to say that we would like to feed our children a Real Food diet but implementing it can seem a formidable challenge. Fear not, we are going to bring them through the process, step by step, just like we are doing for ourselves. This isn't a reality only for those obnoxious mommy bloggers on Instagram, this is a viable target that we can all achieve if we just set up a system and stick with it.

We have to get our kids off this track. We love them dearly, and yet we are making their life so much more difficult. We want them to have fun, and be happy, and we can ensure that by making sure they have a nice stable energy throughout the day. The Happy Buzz is especially happy for a kid. A happy kid can get up without trouble in the morning after getting adequate sleep, they are able to go through the morning routine with little irritation or dragging. They can sit in school and concentrate on what their teacher is helping them learn that day. They can get through the day without any tantrums or tears. Finally, they can go to bed, properly worn out from a full day of learning, growing and new experiences, feeling confident in themselves for being able to manage.

There's just one little snag.

As we learned in Step 3, Fake Food is hard to quit—especially sugar. Kids never asked to get addicted to the white stuff, and yet it is essential that they ditch their habit. How do we do this? Well, I think we do it as gently and painlessly as possible. They will follow along the same steps as we are following to get their Happy buzz. First, we will start adding fruits and vegetables to their diets. You might be thinking that your child will never touch a vegetable. They will, and even more, they will like it. Below, we will go through the steps, but this time with a focus on how to help your kids transition alongside the rest of the family.

Step 1 – One Fruit, One Veg, One Glass of Water per Day

Fruit seems to be an easy sell with children. They already like bananas, apples, and berries. Keep encouraging them to eat those as healthy treats. If they don't like fruit, then follow the same steps as we use with vegetables. It is of utmost importance to get them to eat lots of different colored foods, and we may have to try a few methods to make it happen.

When adding more vegetables into your child's diet, we want to start with what they already like. If they already have a few veg in rotation, then stick with them and add up how many servings they are having per day. We want them in the 6-8 servings every day. Meaning 1-2 veg per meal, with a piece of fruit or two added in as snacks or as a dessert. When you are planning your meals, involve your kids as much as possible. Instead of asking them what they'd like, give them two or three options to pick from. Do this for every meal, and also when packing their lunch. Better yet, get them involved by having them help pack their own lunch while providing a few options they can pick out. This sense of control gives them ownership over their food and will help make them likelier to like their choice. Our brains our wired so that once we commit to a decision, out loud, we want to like our decision and will go out of our way to make that happen. So, an example conversation before you start cooking.

You: "I'm just about to make dinner. I have carrots, peas or a salad I can make up for our vegetable dish. Which would you prefer?"

Child: I guess, carrots would be okay.

You: "Great choice, I was hoping you'd pick carrots. Would you like me to add any toppings to your carrots like butter, parmesan cheese, or salt?"

Child: "Butter, but can I put it on myself?"

You: "Sure, no problem."

By having a conversation with your child that allows them to not only choose their own vegetable, but choose it for the entire family, you are guiding your child in taking responsibility for their healthy eating. When you get to the table, the adults can reiterate how delicious the carrots are, and praise your child for making a great decision. If you have multiple children, let them take turns, or you can make more than one veggie per meal. Heating up frozen vegetables doesn't take long, and most nutritionists say frozen produce can be even healthier than fresh since the farmers flash freeze their crop as soon as it's picked. Fresh veg is also great, but don't get overwhelmed trying to make fancy side dishes, unless you love doing that sort of thing. Another great thing about frozen vegetables is they usually come already diced up and peeled, making it very easy for even the littlest of eaters to indulge without having to spend a large amount of time cutting everything into tiny bites.

"Wait, wait, wait," I can hear some of you saying. "My child would not pick ANY of those vegetables. She'd say no to all three, won't change her mind, and this won't work in our house." I hear you! I don't want to pretend that this method works 100% of the time in my house either. However, this is a fight worth having. It may turn into a battle of the wills, but you are the adult, and you will win. Your child can't drive to the grocery store and pick out an alternate dinner, her only option is what you make her to eat. So, let's say she won't pick a vegetable the first time you try this method. Here's what you do: ask her again calmly, and tell her that if she doesn't pick, then you will pick. However, if you pick, she will need to eat whatever you place in front of her. When you sit down for the meal, set the table with some flavor enhancers she can choose as a topping. Soy Sauce, Cheese, Butter, Salt, and tasty things like that. When you serve her the meal, show her all the add-ins that you have out, and make a game of trying a bite with each different ingredient. Let's say you made carrots anyways. Together, try a bite with parmesan cheese sprinkled on top and rate it. Then try with butter. Then with salt. Then with soy sauce and keep going until all your toppings have been tasted. Then talk about which one was best, which was worse, maybe two could be mixed to make it really tasty. Salt is a huge flavor enhancer, and when your children aren't eating processed food, they can salt their food quite liberally without causing issues. Even in the transition phase, when they're eating both, I think it's okay to let them salt their veg if it gets them to eat it. You can bring the amount down once they are used to eating lots of healthy produce. Remember, in this first step we aren't changing anything else in their diet. We are only ADDING more fruit and veggies.

Another thing we are going to help them with is transitioning from any type of sugary drink to water. This tends to be much easier. If your child only drinks juice, give them the juice and slowly dilute with water until there is just a touch of juice in their drink. Then eventually serve them plain water. If your child complains, then offer them the watered-down juice or plain water; they'll most likely take the watered down juice even if annoyed. Some parents try to get the fruit infusion water bottles and take other fancy routes to get their kids to stop drinking juice. It's your decision, of course, but I would suggest having an end goal of them drinking pure water. Kids need a lot of liquid to stay hydrated throughout the day and cutting up fruit each time they want a drink seems a lot of trouble. It's much easier to just transition them into drinking water, and once they've made the switch, don't buy another bottle of juice. No matter what. Just stick to water as their primary thirst quencher and don't look back.

Step 2: Protein Power

Protein gives people a nice steady buzz of energy, including children. Not only does it help us with our Happy Buzz, but it's an essential building block of a growing body. We need to get our kids into the habit of eating this important nutrient at every meal and snack. Take a look at the list of protein ideas in Step 2 and ask your child what food they find appealing. Be sure to have plenty of options on hand for these little eaters as they can be picky. Each meal of the day should contain a substantial amount of protein for their growing brains and body. Eggs at breakfast is a natural choice. Some sort of meat and/or nuts included in their lunch and dinner will help you meet your goal. As with the previous step, let them help pick out their own food, and offer suggestions on how you can take an old family favorite and make it better by creating it with Real Food only. Do you have pizza every Friday night? Find a recipe using a healthier base and make your own. Throw in some chicken wings and baked apples topped with whipped cream for dessert. Now, your child still feels like they are having the fun family night, but without the Fake Food weighing them down. Pinterest and a basic google search will help you find countless ways to revamp your child's favorite foods using Real ingredients.

Step 3: Cut the Junk

Cutting out sugar and processed foods is very important to teach your kids how to eat for energy. I highly recommend explaining to them why you are making such a change to their diet. Children love to have energy, they love feeling fast, strong and clever. Use these factors to your advantage when explaining to them why you are changing their food choices. When they want a big bowl of sugar-laden cereal for breakfast, explain that you have learned that eating cereal makes their day at school difficult, so we are going to be eating a new breakfast that will help them concentrate while in class, and also have lots of power and energy when they are outside playing. Tell them that by eating this new breakfast, they will be able to run faster, and they will be able to listen to their teacher more easily. Children want to grow. They want to please the adults in their life. Acknowledge their effort, and frame healthy eating as a way to make this process much easier. You aren't punishing them by taking away their favorite sweets, you are teaching them how to eat so that they can do their very best in every new task they try. However, while we know the end goal, how do we wean them off the fake food? Let's look at an example below to see how we can transform breakfast from a sugary, processed disaster to a real food, energy giving power meal.

Kids love waffles. They love the look, the texture, and the thought of pouring a jug of syrup over the top. Let's take their excitement for these sugary cakes and learn how to revamp them into a healthier meal full of produce + protein.

- Banana Waffles

- 1 Banana

- 3 Eggs

- ¼ Cup Oatmeal

- ¼ tsp Vanilla Extract

- Dash of cinnamon

- Tbsp honey/maple syrup/agave syrup/coconut sugar is preferred due to the slow absorption rate (to be phased out once they are used to eating Real Food)

- Blend all ingredients together. Heat up a Belgian waffle iron. Pour batter into waffle iron and cook until waffle looks cooked and is starting to brown in parts. Note, this may take longer to cook than normal waffles due to the banana and eggs.

- Makes 2 large waffles.

To save time in the morning, multiply the batch and freeze the waffles for a later use. Reheat by toasting or placing under the broiler for 5 minutes per side.

Okay, so we have a waffle recipe that looks like it will give our kids the Happy Buzz. You make these up, and it's time to serve the kids. The first time you serve these, set the table with all the typical accoutrements. Syrup, butter, whipped cream; whatever you normally eat with your waffles. Let the kids top their waffles however they normally would, even if that means the plate is swimming in syrup. Now, the next time you serve the waffles, instead of giving the kids free reign over the syrup, pour some into a small ramekin or other portioned serving size bowl. Let them use as much as they'd like out of the ramekin, but no more. The following breakfast, half the amount of syrup in the ramekin and add berries or another fruit into the ramekin. Keep going until you have a ramekin filled with fruit that has been barely coated in syrup. Then take the syrup out altogether. Serve the waffles with sliced fruit only. At this point, your children will be eating eggs, fruit and a little oatmeal for their breakfast before school. Not too bad. From there, we can switch this breakfast to a fun weekend breakfast and try to make their breakfast even less sweet. Scrambled eggs and cheese mixed with leftover meat and veg have become our go-to breakfasts before school. It changes every day and ensures they are filled with protein for energy, and keeps hunger at bay until lunch time. It takes a solid ten minutes to prepare every morning, but it's well worth the effort, when your children are thriving at school.

Besides sugary meals, we must contend with sugary, processed snacks. Kids are constantly growing, and hopefully, constantly moving. Their food intake needs will differ from adults due to their lifestyle and their ever-growing bodies. Snacks are okay, if they aren't too close to mealtimes. Just as with adults, kids need a produce + protein if we want them to maintain their Happy Buzz. With a little forethought and prep, you can make snack time just as easy as opening a packet of chips. Here are some easy kid snacks or light meals:

- Smoked Salmon + Soy Sauce + Cucumbers

- Peanut Butter + Apples + Celery

- Cheese + Pears

- Hard Boiled Egg + Salt + Carrot Sticks

- Sweet Potato disc + Melted Cheese + Pepperoni

- Salted nuts + olives

- Dark Chocolate covered pumpkin seeds + Cherries

- Beef Jerky + Bell Pepper

- Parmesan Chips + Marinara sauce

It's best to time your own step of clearing the house of fake food and sync it with when you think your children are ready to make the leap. Once you throw the fake food out, don't be tempted to buy any more.

Step 4: Get moving; preferably outdoors

While study after study shows that adults are not moving enough, we know that kids are way behind on outdoor fun. There are many reasons for this: the overwhelming enticement of television and screens, the fear of letting our children roam in a dangerous world, the lack of access to a play area. The list could go on, but we all have a good idea of why our children aren't outdoors playing all day like we'd prefer. Diet makes up the overwhelming reason that people, including kids, are overweight, with exercise being a much smaller reason. However, in this book, we aren't looking at weight, we are looking at energy, and this can be used as a great motivation to get your kids moving.

For adults, I recommend getting your physical activity outdoors for mental health reasons. Something about being out in the elements gives people a much bigger boost of energy and mental clarity than staring at a television screen in the gym. For youngsters, this is even more important. Young children learn so much just by being outside. They learn textures, sounds, seasons, and can get dirty. They can strengthen their imagination by being forced to play in the wild, instead of with toys that dictate the type of activity they do. They build up their immune system by coming into contact with so many different materials. Try to schedule at least an hour of playtime outdoors every day. If you have a back garden, set up a safe parameter to allow some unsupervised exploration—even for the little ones. Send all the kids out to play while you're making dinner at night. Let the older ones learn to watch out for the younger ones. If you don't have a back garden, bring them to a playground. Encourage their school or nursery to provide adequate outdoor activities for the children. Try to get them outside as much as your schedule allows, and you will see the positive impact on their energy levels, their sleep schedules, and their level of happiness.

Another great habit to form is a family stroll. If you work all day, this may seem like a big undertaking, but it's worth it, I promise. If you work, and feel your nights turn into chaos, you might abhor the idea of adding in another 20-minute activity every day. Yet, with a little planning, you'll see that it can either set the tone for a much calmer evening and become a good way to wind down a hectic day before bedtime activities. Try taking a stroll around the neighborhood as soon as you arrive home. Use this time to reconnect and discard any stresses from the day before entering the evening. Another option is to take a walk after dinner to help your food digest and allow the kids to get that last burst of energy out before bedtime. When and where you go, don't matter as much as the act of forming the new habit of time outdoors everyday.

Step 5: Sleep

When my first child was born, her pediatrician was an older man, who had several children of his own. Every new mom's worry was quickly pacified by a quick phone call to this doctor who had seen it all, not only at work, but with his own, now grown, children. He was of the mindset that children were designed to fall, designed to withstand the nervous parent, and designed to grow, no matter the circumstances. His calm and easy-going attitude towards rearing children had a great soothing effect on a very anxious mother.

However, one thing our doctor did take very seriously was sleep. At every checkup or appointment, he would want to know the amount of hours the baby was sleeping, and this continued for our entire time with him. One time I asked him why he was so laid back about most other matters but seemed to be so strict with sleep. He started telling me about how frustrated he got hearing about these new parents allowing the kids to set their own bedtimes, and that the most well-meaning parents, those who buy everything organic, go to all the baby classes, read all the books (In other words, very involved and loving parents), were utterly failing on sleep routines for their kids, and he believed the effect on development was a big cause for concern. He pointed out that, while different children have different sleep needs, it is always better to error on the side of too much sleep, rather than too little, and in today's world, there were a lot of children getting too few hours of shut eye.

Think about what happens if you go for a few days where you only got five hours of sleep each night. You can manage, but you will probably be tired, cranky, struggling to focus, perhaps having mood swings. Children function the same way, but they don't know they're having a hard time due to fatigue. They might nod off in the car after an after school activity, but you will rarely find a child asking to go up to bed. It's up to us, as the parents, to make sure they are getting the right amount of sleep each night and teaching them the importance of doing so. Having a wind-down routine and sticking to a bedtime, can help them train their brains on how to go to sleep.

Amount of Sleep Needed by Age:

0-12 months old: 14-16 hours per day (including naps)

1-3 years old: 12-14 hours per day (including naps)

4-6 years old: 10-12 hours per day

7-12 years old: 10-11 hours per day

12-18 years old: 8-9 hours per day

Just as with adults, take the time they need to wake up and count backwards to figure out the time they need to be asleep by. If you have a 5-year-old that needs to be up at 7am for school, then they need to be asleep between 7-9pm. Try to err on the longer side, especially if your child is active. At least thirty minutes before bed, turn the living space into a quiet zone. Dim lights, no electronics, quiet and calm. Use the time to read books, or get dressed, or play a quiet game. Do the same routine each night and stay consistent on bedtime.

The Mess-Ups

Occasionally, your child will be in a situation where fake food is unavoidable. It's up to you to decide how you will maneuver in that situation. But, if you can transform your child's diet to 95% real food, I don't believe in feeling guilty over some bad meals here and there. They are going to be invited to birthday parties, playdates, and family gatherings where other people are eating very tempting food to a child. If they are little and you are serving their plate, try to balance out the fake food with a few real food options. If they're older, hopefully they have been taught to make healthy choices. However, if they go hog wild, eat all the fake food in sight, then use the subsequent meltdown, tiredness and irritability as a teachable moment. The next day just have a small conversation about how their food choices contributed to how they felt, and then leave them to think about it on their own. Hopefully, by the time they are an adult you will have passed onto them a firm connection between food and energy, and they will be able to make wise decisions, but children usually learn the hard way, and there's no need to be militant. I say this to give you permission to not only mess up yourself, but also with your kids and not feel guilty. We live in a society filled with fake food, and other alluring objects. You will not be the perfect parent. Cut yourself some slack. When you get off course, reroute yourself towards real food and outdoor time, and you'll get back on track. Use those times as a learning opportunity for young kids, and you will be setting your children up for a Happy Buzz for life.

Tips and Tricks

- As you, the adult, quit your addiction to Fake Food and start to incorporate a healthy mindset into your life, bring your children on the same journey. This diet is for the entire family and can be done as a unit.

- Point out the positive changes occurring in their lives due to the Happy Buzz. If they used to have a meltdown every evening and those start to become rare, praise them for their positive change, and explain how their healthy eating habits have allowed them to shine. If they used to complain when it was time for the family walk, but now get their shoes on and look forward to it, remind them of how far they've come, and how great it feels to be outdoors. Help them to realize that being outside is more fun than sitting on the couch watching cartoons.

- Look for teachable moments in situations to contrast their new behavior with the old. Positive reinforcement will help them rewire their own brains to appreciate the differences between feeling full of power and energy, and slow and lethargic. Kids love to feel powerful, so remind them as often as possible how they are in control of how their bodies feel.

- Give your children as much input as you feel they are ready to handle—from helping with grocery shopping to planning, or preparing their school lunches. This will allow their self confidence to grow in their decision-makin skills.

Above all, use this opportunity to grow closer together by sharing a common goal, and enjoying the life changing benefits of Real Food, the outdoors, and great sleep. The entire family will be happier for it.

Real Food can be Fast Food

There's a misconception about eating a Real Food diet, and it goes like this:

"I know I shouldn't be eating all this fast food and junk food, but I just don't have time to cook."

There are variations on this mantra, where the excuse can also be not knowing how to cook, with some people believing they can't even boil water. If this is you, the time for excuses has come and gone. You are going to have to learn a few basics around the kitchen. Whether you want to take your knowledge into amateur chef level, is up to you, but you at least need to know how to prepare a few things that will nourish your body. Humans have been feeding themselves without Fake Food for millions of years, and with a lot more hardship, so you can learn how to prepare a few things. In our rewired brain, we need to convince it of another reality. There are no more fast food restaurants, no more frozen dinners, no more pop tarts for breakfast. All of those locations have been destroyed, and they are not available anymore. If you want to eat, you are going to have to gather some Real Food and figure out a way to put it together. In the chapter on Protein, there is a list of snack ideas that only require simple preparation, such as washing and slicing a vegetable or fruit, and pairing it with a protein. You can always eat a larger portion of these pairings and use that as a meal. However, if you enjoy sitting down at the table and delving into a hot meal, then a few basic tips can help your cooking skills improve quickly.

Salt is essential

Salt gets a bad rap since we consume too much by way of Fake Food. However, when we eat a diet of Real Food, we can use salt liberally without too much risk. Obviously, ask your doctor if you have any medical conditions that might prevent you from eating salt. For everybody else, salt is your friend. Salt is the reason that food tastes so much better when eating out. Chef's know the importance of seasoning and tend to always have a salt tub nearby when cooking. When preparing meat, salt is the number one thing that will make it taste good. No matter if you are making steak or chicken, grab a big pinch of salt and rub it into every crevice on the surface of the meat.

Roasting vs. Pan Frying

Let the meat come to room temperature before cooking, and then throw in the pan for a quick fry (this method works well for flat pieces of meat such as steak or pork chops). Or put the meat in a roasting pan and pop in the oven. These are the two easiest methods of preparing meat without much hassle. If you only have twenty minutes to get dinner out, then pan frying is going to be much quicker, so choose your meal accordingly. If you have time to let something sit and cook in the oven, roasting tends to be an easier method, as once it's in the oven, you can just leave it there to cook, while you do other things. You can also make a larger amount of this type of meat and save the extra for meals later. Another benefit of roasting meat is you can easily line the bottom of the roasting dish with vegetables to serve alongside the meat. The juices from the meat will drip onto the vegetables to add some extra flavor. If you are feeling extra adventurous, add some dollops of butter onto the veg so that the butter and meat juice will all melt together making the vegetables taste extra indulgent.

Meal Prep

There is a lot of information out there on meal prep. I understand why this works for some people. You spend a Sunday afternoon washing, chopping and cooking up a large volume of food. Then pack it away into containers that you can grab and take with you later on in the week. This is a great idea for those out and about all day. However, eating the same meal every day can be too boring for some people and trigger them to go for fast food instead of sticking to their meal plan. If that's you, then recognize that meal prepping isn't really for you. Instead of pre-packaged meals, use this idea for your fridge instead. Wash and cut all your produce and place into clear containers in the refrigerator, where you can mix and match depending on what you are in the mood for. Think, fresh berries, cucumber slices, carrot sticks, salty nuts, brown rice cooked and cooled, lettuce and leafy greens, cooked meat, cheese, butter, sauces, cream, and more. Then when you are packing your lunch, combine as you wish. Use the veg and meat in an easy egg scramble, or in a salad, or just eat separately if you really don't have the time to make anything.

Weeknight Family Dinners

If the entire family is working and at school all day, then dinnertime can feel extremely rushed and stressful. The best way to overcome this hurdle is to make a meal plan for the week. This can be as fancy or as simple as you like. If you eat the same dinner every Tuesday night, does it really matter? If it works, it works. Don't overcomplicate things unless you have the time and desire. At the very least, have a list of five meals that you can make and make well. The best list allows for different circumstances. One meal may be a crock pot meal you can put together in during the morning and have piping hot and ready to eat for those days when you need to have food ready as soon as you walk in the door at night. Have a meal that you can assemble on a sheet pan and throw in the oven, while you get other things done without fussing over the food. Have a meal that can be made in a pan by just adding more and more ingredients. Have a no-cook meal for hot days, or days when you just aren't in the mood for cooking at all. And have a family favorite that everybody loves and is worth the extra time and effort. With your list of meals in hand, decide what your schedule is for the day or week, and decide which meal fits your time frame the best. If you have an early day, make a more elaborate meal on that day, and make twice as much, freezing the extra for a day when you are booked solid. Once you have your list, see if there are ways you can vary those meals for a new meal using the same technique.

The Five Meal Plan

Crock Pot Dinner: Cheap cuts work best. Get a roast of some type, chop some onions and garlic for the bottom, lay the roast on top and season with salt and pepper. Add extra dried herbs and spice or spice mixes for more flavor. Preboil or roast potatoes or sweet potatoes that you can quickly heat up on the side, along with some frozen vegetables.

Sheet Pan Dinner: Chicken Thighs laid on top of summer or winter squash, baked until chicken is cooked through. A meal like this can be assembled the night beforeand popped into the oven as soon as you get home.

Stove Top Meal: Sautee diced ham and bell peppers until cooked and heated through. In a separate bowl, scramble eggs with milk, and pour the mixture over the ham and peppers, stirring until cooked through. Serve with a side salad.

No-Cook Meal: Mixed Greens, topped with loads of chopped vegetables, cheese, and meats. Serve with a variety of dressings.

Family Favorite: Your choice.

In this example, you have five meals you can throw together easily, given the type of day you're having. Once you have these locked down, you can easily swap some ingredients for more variety. Let's say you are making a slow cooker recipe. Normally, you slice some onions, carrots and bell peppers, and salt a beef roast the night before work. In the morning, you throw it all into the slow cooker with some butter, and a BBQ seasoning for extra flavor. When you get home, throw together a simple salad and serve. The next week, you can use the same method, but instead of beef, you get a pork roast. If you are craving Thai this week, instead of a BBQ blend, you'll add chilis, shallots, garlic, and whole sweet potatoes with your favorite Thai spice blend. Get home, add lettuce wraps, sliced cucumber and carrot, and your favorite condiments on the side. Now you have two completely different meals, using the same technique and taking the same amount of time. This way of planning will help eliminate feeling overwhelmed when trying to determine what to cook during a busy week. You will always have a few staples you can throw together in a rush.

Mistakes Were Made

There you are, going about your day, eating real foods, feeling powerful and happy, and all the sudden.... A pint of ice cream jumped out and poured itself into your mouth!!! The horror! You didn't even see it coming. Now, we all know that didn't really happen, but the way some people talk about their diet, you would almost believe that Fake Food was just forcing its way into their mouths without any input from the person themselves. While an addiction to Fake Food can make us feel powerless to the allure of a sugary or processed food, we need to take some accountability over who is in charge here. This isn't to say that we need to beat ourselves up when we mess up, but we do need to acknowledge that we have gone off course, and self-correct.

If you have switched over to a Real Food diet and find yourself in a vulnerable situation, there's a chance that you may abandon your clean, healthy eating strategy and partake in your old ways. We are creatures of habit, and we have a much easier time sticking to a routine than having new experiences every day. Once you get out of your normal schedule, be aware that you are in a vulnerable spot in regard to your new way of eating. There are many situations that we may find ourselves in that make us feel that we must resort to our old ways. You may be travelling and find yourself stuck in the airport, or on a long flight, and decide to grab fast food instead of a salad. Due to how expensive Real Food is at airports, you might not even have a choice. Once you are on the plane, there is a good chance you won't even have a choice to eat Real Food. It will be Fake Food or nothing.

Maybe you just met a new set of friends and have decided to get dinner together. You've always had social anxiety, and the thought of making conversation with strangers is already stressful, without the added pressure of needing to navigate an unknown menu. Instead of thinking about what will give your body the Happy Buzz, you are more tempted to order a sugary cocktail followed by pizza buzz. How do we handle these new situations successfully?

There are two options. We either give in to the temptation and eat the fake food, or we persevere with our quest to feel good, and figure out a way to still eat Real Food, even in uncharted territory. If you are going on a trip and need to fly there, you have a few ways to manage this situation and keep on track. You can pack a lunch to bring with you. Bring some fruit, veggies, and protein with you to the airport. This will also save you some money. Likewise, when going out to eat, you can plan ahead to save yourself from having to make any last-minute bad decisions. Most restaurants have their menus posted online, and you can go through and pick out your meal before you even leave the house. But let's say you didn't do that and for whatever reason, you messed up. You ate the Fake Food, you skipped your walk, you went to bed way too late, whatever. You might be experiencing guilt, frustration, tiredness, mood swings, and feeling like a big failure. What do you do now? You are back to feeling like crap, and unmotivated. I'll tell you what we do when we backslide into this situation. Are you ready? Pay attention here, because this is very important.

All we need to do is acknowledge we messed up, and then get back to the steps that lead us to the Happy Buzz.

That's it? Yep, we aren't here to harangue ourselves and feed into negative self-talk. You messed up? Who cares? You're a flawed human being; it happens. All that matters is what happens after your mistake. Do you wallow in it for a week of energy sucking behavior, or do you pop back up and get back on schedule? You pop back up.

Yes, you have just made things more difficult for yourself; you might be more tired, you might have a difficult time getting out the door for your walk, but you can do it. You've already done it before, so, of course, you can do it again. Acknowledging that this was a fluke, and not your normal, will help your brain separate what is an anomaly versus what is a habit. A little while ago, eating eight servings of produce every day may have been an anomaly, but now, that is your normal. You have already made the change. Eating Fake Food is now strange and unusual for your brain. Remind yourself of how much you enjoy getting out in nature, and just go. Don't overthink it. Just start the process of going. Get dressed, put your hiking shoes on, grab your keys, walk to the door. If you've been staying up until crazy hours and have thrown off your sleep schedule, make a point not to nap or sleep in, and then adhere to your bedtime. At some point in this ritual, your brain will go from resistance mode, into habit mode. It will recognize the pattern and start acting accordingly. You just need to force yourself to take the first steps.

While messing up on sleep or exercise can be frustrating and set you back in terms of energy, messing up on your diet can be a bit trickier. Since our diet is the main source of energy in the Happy Buzz equation, we need to make sure we stick to eating Real Foods. As discussed in Step 3, when you mess up on your diet, especially with eating Fake Food, it can be tough to get back into gear. When you eat processed junk, especially sugar laden garbage, it can reactivate your addiction and send you into a spiral. You may have gone six months without touching the white stuff, and then have a slice of cake, and you will feel as if no time has passed. If this happens, throw out the remaining Fake Food, and get right back on track. If you are finding it difficult, then start back at Step 1, and go through the process again. This time it should be much quicker than the initial endeavor since you have already made it a habit in your brain. You may be able to go right back into Step 3 and start there. No matter where you need to start, just get back into the process and keep going.

Conquering an addiction is an enormously difficult goal to achieve. As with any other addiction, the journey to being clean can be a pull and tug to get through to the other side. That's okay. It might take you multiple rounds to finally have beaten the beast. Instead of beating yourself up for failures, recognize that every time you persevere and get back on that horse, you are building fortitude and strength. It will pay off, if you keep trying until you succeed.

Energy = Happiness

Those who have made it through the steps and have committed to finding new ways to enhance their newfound energy have most certainly solved one of life's most sought after questions: what is happiness, and am I happy? You may not have realized it yet, but you will as you continue on your journey.

Happiness is one of those esoteric ideas that we all at once understand, yet also fail to define. It can mean different things to different people, one might feel that contentment marks a happy life. Another might feel that pursuing pleasure leads to happiness. Financial success is thought to bring happiness to a dreary life. There is one thing that all these thoughts have in common; without energy, they will never come to fruition. It's impossible to be content if you are in a constant struggle to get out of bed. Those who love to indulge in pleasure will never be able to fully experience the hedonistic delights if they don't have the energy to go where the fun is. For certain, financial success does not come to the lethargic.

Whichever path you choose to pursue to achieve your life's goals, you need energy, and lots of it, to enjoy yourself and be happy. Whether trying to start a new business, to deciding to have children, to mustering the courage to travel somewhere new and exotic, energy is needed to see your dreams through. Without adequate energy, you are left with brilliant ideas never realized, locations never explored, and lives that were pondered, but not fully lived. The path to happiness starts with energy.

As with all journeys in life, it is easy to get side-tracked and end up in a place you didn't intend to visit. My hope with this book is that it is a simple guide to navigate you back to a Happy Buzz, no matter how many times you need to use it. I tried to make it short and sweet, so that you, dear reader, can use it as a handy tool to kickstart your life and make the most of your precious few years on Earth. I hope it changes your life in the same way that is has changed mine.

I wish you the best of luck and hope that you feel better than you have ever felt before. I hope you are able to shake off the Fake Food addiction and go on to lead the life you are meant to lead, once full of success, joy, and a Happy Buzz.

Good Luck and God Speed.

www.ingramcontent.com/pod-product-compliance
Lightning Source LLC
Chambersburg PA
CBHW070737250726
48662CB00004B/1570